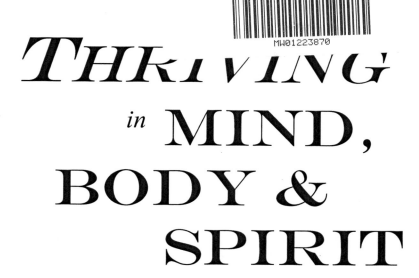

THRIVING
in MIND,
BODY &
SPIRIT

Awakening to God's Truths and Promises

Dearest Debbie Nov 3rd/07
I wish you the
best that God has Victory
to offer you.
in Christ
Shaun

Dr. Shaun Dyler

Outskirts Press, Inc.
Denver, Colorado

CONTENTS

ACKNOWLEDGMENTS

I want to acknowledge first that God, the center of my life, is my source of strength, wisdom, peace, and joy.

I would like to express my love and admiration for my wife, Katy, my best friend and partner in life. She inspired me to make this book a reality. Several years ago, Katy gave me a journal. She believed that I had to share my knowledge of medicine and my faith in God to help others. This began my commitment to the process of writing this book, and I am profoundly grateful to her even though the process has been difficult, time consuming, and frustrating at times.

I would also like to extend my gratitude to all of the teachers in my life, including my parents whom I love dearly, my relatives, and my patients. A special thank you goes to my good friend Carolyn Wood who helped me put some of my scattered thinking into words and who always challenged me on the biblical accuracy of this book. My good friend Barbara Tuttle who pays attention to all the fine details and no less special is my thank you to my most recent editor Mike Umlandt, whose expertise and professionalism have made the book as polished as it appears to you.

Finally, my thanks to God for my daughter and son, who bring me joy I never imagined possible. Tatiana and Alexander help me realize how precious life truly is and teach me to keep laughing like a child (and adult) should.

INTRODUCTION

I have searched for and sought after truth most of my life. I wanted to know the truth concerning deep philosophical questions such as "What is the purpose of being?" and "Why is there so much suffering in the world?" I also wanted to know the medical truth regarding why my grandma got cancer, why my other grandma developed diabetes, and why I suffered from acne.

I have always been a serious student of life. I have sought for answers in both Western and Eastern medicine and in Western and Eastern religions and philosophies. My journey, which continues, has had ups and downs. As the result of struggling with my own health, however, I have found answers for many individuals' health problems.

More importantly, I believe I have also found most, if not all, of the answers in my search for purpose and meaning. The principles in this book can improve your life significantly and in some cases dramatically.

Some people would say that I have become religious and narrow-minded, and suggested that I'd sell a lot more books if I left the spiritual part out. My objective for writing this book, however, is not to sell a lot of copies; it is to help as many people as possible achieve optimal health—mentally, physically, and spiritually. It's been a challenge to share what I believe to be completely true without sounding self-righteous and perhaps diminishing what others believe to be true. I have tried to avoid this, but inevitably fail at times. My only request to you, the reader, is that you read this book with an open heart and an inquiring mind, and that ultimately you examine your own thought systems, habits, and patterns.

As a naturopathic physician and acupuncturist, I have seen many individuals who have enjoyed good physical health but still suffered from depression, anxiety, and a sense of vulnerability. I have also seen individuals with poor physical health and yet who had a deep joy and unwavering faith. It's been my joy to help them understand their bodies better. Simple chemical, hormonal, and nutritional imbalances were quite often the cause of their poor health.

For my patients who were fairly healthy physically and yet suffered psychologically, I still found the need to address some chemical imbalances, but more important was the need to address their minds and spirits. Many self-help books attempt to address some of these issues, but I have never found a book that clearly and effectively tied them all together. This is what I have attempted to do in this book, and it has certainly been a challenge. I will probably always feel that I could have written it better or explained things differently, but after six years of revisions and additions, I have decided to bring you what I have.

Wherever you are in your own journey toward wellness and whatever you believe spiritually, I hope that my experiences and beliefs will challenge and inspire you to make changes in your life. This book is geared for the individual who is searching for answers on how to live a better life. If you are already at peace and joyful most of the time, sleep well at night, have excellent physical health, and are confident that you're on your way to heaven, then this book is probably not for you.

If you already have faith in God, great! If you read this book, I believe you'll gain insights into improving your health and living the abundant life that God promises.

If you are not a believer or believe differently than I do, I hope and pray that you examine seriously what I have written and, more importantly, what God says in His Word. Regardless, I hope you will benefit from the health principles in this book.

I have seen the benefits, in my life and in hundreds of patients, of properly addressing all of the aspects of our being—our minds, bodies, and spirits. Occasionally I have witnessed miraculous results, but most of the time I see people beginning to apply the principles I teach in this book and as a result become empowered to make the daily choices necessary for optimal health. I am not perfect and need to rely on these same principles each and every day as well. My success comes when I rely on the strength, wisdom, power, love, mercy, and grace of God.

CHAPTER 1
Awakening to the Truth

1.1 Life Is Difficult...but God!
(The undeserved grace, mercy, and favor that God pours out on His children)

Just when life feels under control, a storm hits.

Picture yourself driving down a beautiful country road on a sunny spring day. You reach to tune in your favorite radio station and it comes in crystal clear. But 10 minutes later, dark clouds appear on the horizon, and the radio snaps and crackles. Fortunately you're still able to hear a weather alert about a tornado in the direction you're driving! You quickly turn around and head for home. Before long the sun is shining again and you're gleefully singing along with the music on the radio.

Are you "tuned in"? You might get tired of hearing me say it, but it's my premise and experience that staying tuned in—tuned in to God—is the key to a meaningful and good life. When we seek God, pray and get to know Him personally, obey and follow His commands, we can live "in tune" with Him. When we are in tune with God we are more likely to make good decisions and thereby avoid a lot of stress and anxiety associated with bad choices. Living in conscious, constant communion with our Creator helps us gain wisdom, insight, and reverence for life that in turn will shape our every choice, both big and small, along the way. You can't allow the static of the world's pressures to distract you from God's voice.

Seek to understand what God is trying to tell you through your challenging circumstances, the people He uses as teachers in life, and the body He created for you. The challenging circumstances in our lives are not haphazard, disjointed events that we fall in and out of. Neither are the people in our lives. Ponder and you may be able to recognize patterns that may be continually repeating themselves. The story line and actors might change but the scenario is familiar if we slip out of denial and connect the dots.

So what are the life lessons? The main life lesson is that we must die to self in order to find life in God. We will explore this in depth in this chapter. Most other lessons will stem from this and will include lessons in our honesty, in our ability to forgive others, in our ability to love others, in our ability to not judge others, and in our ability to admit wrongs. Is everything in life a lesson? No. There are also life reminders, life tests, and spiritual warfare. There may be reminders about the consequences of our bad choices, reminders about the fragility of life here on earth, and reminders that we are not in control of most variables other then our choice of how we react and respond to people and circumstances in our life. Then there are the tests to see if we have learned the life lessons, the tests to see if we have truly died to our self, and the tests to see if we have our priorities in life correct. And finally there is spiritual warfare for our heart, mind, and present peace/joy. This staying tuned in also applies to our bodies. Health issues and chronic symptoms are also trying to get our attention, calling us to dig deeper into understanding the root of the problem. Learn everything you can about your body and how it works (see Chapter 4). Pay attention to your body's warning signals—an ounce of prevention is truly better than a pound of cure!

Tuning in to God is a daily, lifetime, moment-to-moment choice that none of us has mastered. We all wish that avoiding the storms of life were as simple as stopping the car and driving the other way. Life is so much bigger than us no matter how hard we wish we were in control. The important question is: How do we find peace, joy, and hope in spite of turbulent weather? There is only one answer to this question. Turn to God!

The storms of life can either knock us off of our weak foundations or propel us to ask the right questions about life and begin to sort out what really matters. A storm is often an opportunity to re-evaluate our philosophies and habits. I know it's easy to shrug off situations as bad luck or coincidence; instead it's critical for us to look for the lessons to learn and apply in our lives. Yes! We are all in the school of life and some lessons are more difficult than others. The rules of life have not changed. God is the same yesterday, today, and forever. The unchanging God, however, uses changing circumstances and people in our lives to try to get our attention to bring about our change. The question is, are we willing to change? Are we willing to learn our lessons? You and I clearly have a choice to make. To continue in the school of denial and pride and learn life lessons the hard way or to become a diligent student—tuning in to God and learning His definition of how to have life and life more abundantly.

A few years ago, as I was wrapping up this manuscript and feeling pretty good about it, my mom called to tell me excitedly she was finally going to get married—officially—to her companion of 20 years. It was difficult for me to hold back my judgmental tendencies since my mom claimed to be a Catholic and yet lived in a common law marriage for two decades and had two children out of wedlock. I did my best and simply hoped she could turn things around and have a clear conscience about her life. Things were far from perfect. Bill, her soon-to-be-husband, suffered from a painful divorce in his past as well and often turned to alcohol to numb some of his own pains and frustrations.

The day leading up to the wedding was filled with both hope and tension around these dynamics. Fortunately the wedding went smoothly, and then there was only the reception to worry about. The loud voices and smell of alcohol were too much for my wife and me, so we said our good-byes at about 9 p.m. As we walked to our hotel across the street, my younger half-brother Steven and I hugged and parted ways, looking forward to an early morning on the golf course.

It was a restless night. The adjacent rooms were occupied by loud, intoxicated partiers, and we tossed and turned in our efforts to get some sleep. At 3:30 a loud pounding on the door awakened us. It was a police officer. A variety of thoughts and situations raced through my mind, but the officer's somber look portrayed terrible news.

"Your brother was involved in a serious car accident."

No other words were necessary. I knew that Steven did not survive.

My life changed in more ways than I realized at the time. Through the tragedy, God not only comforted me but also opened my eyes to see how serious life is, how daily thoughts and actions can lead to life or death (physically, emotionally, or spiritually), and how the battle for my mind and heart is very real. I began to develop spiritual boldness, discernment, and a heart to share the truth of God's goodness to all of my friends, family, and whoever else was willing to listen.

Going Deeper with God

I was drawn to go deeper with God and eventually with this book. Before losing my brother, my book was shaping up to be a positive, feel-good message, but it lacked depth and important truths. God had allowed me to go through this tragedy so that I would be more real with Him, with myself, and with anyone I would interact with, including you, the reader.

The spiritual concepts of this book are universal truths that I have embraced as a true believer. I am privileged to have the Bible as my life manual, and I have done my best to be biblically correct.

Much of what I talk about, especially in the chapter on physical health (Chapter 4), is scientifically valid and backed by research. Some of the things that I say may not be proven scientifically, but I have found them to be valid and true based on my own physical healing journey and that of hundreds of clients.

4

A Better Life

Most people I know want to live a better, more fulfilling life. The question is, what does that better life look like? America is currently the most prosperous nation in the world and yet we have the highest rate of depression, divorce, and burn out. Our pop culture media idolize youthfulness, celebrity lifestyles, fast and endless money, consumerism, sexual freedom, and total acceptance of fringe behavior. Our media and current culture actually reward bad behavior, praise outrageous attitudes, encourage ego-driven pursuits, and look down upon traditional values that ensure the success and longevity of any society. Young girls are encouraged to claim their womanhood through overt sexuality, and young boys are lost in their search for role models. Double-income parents willingly outsource the care of their kids in order to pursue the bigger house and more toys. Marriages are trivialized through the shows that parade on television, and unless we wake up the traditional family is going to become a small minority at best. We have lost our sense of purpose and community. All the modern technological advances in many ways have pushed us back further into our cocoons. The world has become a global village and yet there is more depravity and loneliness than ever. Our problem does not appear to be global warming; it appears to be global cooling! A lack of connection and real meaning in life. We were created for so much more than things. We were created with purpose for a purpose and will constantly search in vain for happiness and satisfaction until we realize this.

Success as defined by the world has nothing to do with the abundant life that God says is a possibility. The abundant life may or may not involve material wealth. At its root is a deep loving relationship with the Creator Himself and with the people in your life. The fruit of living a life that puts God first is what we all desire: love, joy, peace, patience, gentleness, goodness, faith, and self-control.

Are you experiencing this kind of life, or are you caught in autopilot mode?

Living on Autopilot

Life on autopilot is simply the result of complacency, fear, ignorance, poor health, or deep family patterns that we all fall prey to. It is a life driven by feelings and emotions, reactions to others, and egocentric motives. I am in no way diminishing the negative impact of past traumas, certain parental traits, and poor physical health. These are all real, valid realities—difficult to identify at times and often even more difficult to treat. However, if we take little or no time to reflect on the past, to gain insight, to observe our own behaviors and patterns, or to seek professional help in order to heal, then by default we follow the path of least resistance. We avoid the challenge of discovering what is best, hoping that we can simultaneously avoid all pain. *Instead, we choose, either consciously or subconsciously, the most painful route through life.*

This is one reason why depression, loneliness, fatigue, and even illness plague so many. Some of us attempt to numb ourselves with alcohol, work, antidepressants, smoking, food, exercise, sex, or even religion. Others may use more subtle techniques to avoid reality and as a result experience low-level misery. Avoidance and denial have never solved a problem, and never will, whether physical, psychological, or spiritual. In regard to medical intervention, there are certainly situations in which prescriptions for antidepressants, sedatives, or painkillers are medically necessary. Nevertheless, the use of medications is now so prevalent that we would have to call most of society "dysfunctional." A spiritual or physical Band-Aid does very little to heal an underlying problem. In Chapter 4, I share with you many natural approaches to deal with common health troubles or "dis-ease" that are safer and in many instances more effective than prescription medications.

Reflection

I strongly encourage you to read this book with two or three other people who are committed to making changes, holding one another accountable, and praying for one another. I would also recommend you keep a journal of your reflections, further questions you may have, and current responses to the questions in this book. Review in six months.

Below are some areas to reflect on to determine if you are operating on autopilot. The autopilot life resembles depression. Understanding and acknowledging if your problem is weighted in the physical, mental/emotional, or spiritual realm can help determine where you most need help. Of course, these three aspects of your being cannot be fully separated, but nonetheless compartmentalizing will be helpful in this application.

Physical signs of the autopilot life:
Low energy, irritability, anxiety, insomnia or oversleep, loss of libido, lack of focus/concentration, overwhelmed easily, recurring infections, cannot assimilate new information easily, have given up on hobbies and regular exercise.

Mental/emotional signs of the autopilot life:
Nostalgic, obsessed with negative thoughts, driven to overwork/overachieve, hopelessness, oversensitivity to other people's problems or emotionally numb, easily cry, lack of laughter, pessimistic/negative, sarcastic.

Spiritual signs of the autopilot life:
Lack of joy, lack of hope, lack of patience, lack of identity/low self-esteem, lack of deep connection with God and people.

1. Are you living on autopilot at least some of the time or perhaps even most of the time? Acknowledging your problem is the first step toward healing. You will find solutions in the respective chapter sections in this book. Denial has never solved a problem and never will!

2. Are you experiencing daily joy? If not, why? Are there areas in your life that are a regular source of stress?

3. Is your body giving you any warning signals that you are

ignoring or covering up with over-the-counter medications?

4. Do you find yourself repeating some of your parents' patterns that were/are dysfunctional?

5. Are you good at putting on a face for others? Are you ready to be transparent and open with those who care most about you?

6. Are there particular circumstances or people in your life that God is using to get your attention? What do you think your lesson, reminder, or test is?

7. Are you taking the time daily to learn more about God and getting to know Him personally?

8. Are you willing to seek the appropriate professional help? Or are your fears and pride going to get in the way?

9. Does talking about spiritual and personal issues make you uncomfortable? Where do you think that stems from?

10. Welcome to the journey toward wellness. The process may have ups and downs, but the fact that you are choosing to face your issues and embrace God's truths and promises already means success!

1.2 Are You Awake?

Through my own awakening process I have realized that I had spent (and still do occasionally) much of my life in a dream, a state of unreality concocted from fears, fantasies, false beliefs or lies, and past traumas.

Pause for a few minutes to consider how your own life is unfolding. Do you ever feel that you are losing control over your life, or that things are not going the way you had hoped or planned?

Do you try to muster up positive thoughts, exercise self-discipline, or follow a careful plan only to find that all of your efforts seem to fall short after a while? Even when life is going as planned, do you sense that something is missing or that everything you have built could crumble at any moment?

This sense of vulnerability, disillusionment, and emptiness is common to all humanity. At its root is a desire to feed and serve our ego. Ego is the sense of self, separate from God. Think of EGO as an acronym for Edging God Out. It is basically the part of us that believes we are the masters of our own destiny, that life is all about us, or on the other extreme that we are insignificant, unplanned beings in this universe. These perceptions stem from our own experiences in life—what we have been taught culturally, our religious upbringing, our past traumas, what we have observed in our parents, how our peers have defined us, and most importantly how we have interpreted all of these life experiences.

Maybe you were the class clown, the skinny boy or the overweight girl, or perhaps the shy child and have yet to overcome the stigma. Perhaps you are putting on a face or image for everyone when in reality you feel insecure, angry, or depressed. If this is you, the good news is that there is hope! Lasting happiness (as opposed to momentary pleasure), contentment, peace, and health only come from knowing God personally and allowing Him to grow, shape, and mold us into the people we were meant to be.

"Awakening" is the process in which we seek to know the truth, discover who God is, and then ultimately surrender ourselves to Him. Being tuned in to God is a part of this awakening process and is critical if we are to thrive in all areas of our lives.

Being tuned in extends into all aspects of our lives. Dietary choices, lifestyle choices, and especially our words and actions can all be brought under God's direction. Being tuned in to God helps us to be aware of our choices. It helps us to more closely observe the environment around us and our feelings, thoughts, and reactions within us. Being tuned in allows us to be aware of the gift of the present moment, thereby not dwelling on the past or living in the future at the expense of the now. When we are awake and tuned in, we can have a clear awareness of our choices—to do things God's way or our own way. We are also better able to discern between good (good, better, and best) and evil. Most importantly, when we are awake and tuned in, we can recognize that we are under God's protection, direction, blessing—and His infinite mercy and grace.

In the awakened state you truly recognize your need for all of these provisions. Your goal in the awakened state is to get to know your Creator better, to seek His will for your life, and to share this Good News with others. He, in turn, promises to provide everything else—the basics such as food, clothing, shelter, and emotional well-being such as peace, joy, and hope. Renewed strength and even wealth are promises that God has made to His people throughout the ages. Does this mean that you will never have challenges—that you'll never contract a disease, struggle to make ends meet, or suffer physical pain? No! If you have never read about the life of Job in the Bible, I recommend you spend an hour with this fascinating book. What Job endured puts all of my struggles in a healthy perspective. The Bible is very clear that we will have problems. *"These things I have spoken to you, that in me you may have peace. In the world you will have tribulation; but be of good cheer, I have overcome the world."*[1]

Ego Is the Problem

All of us are good at putting on a face for one another. We may even appear to be doing well when in fact our lives are falling apart. I have been there, and perhaps you have too. Maybe it's financial troubles. Perhaps it is marriage troubles, anxiety, or depression? It could be addiction to drugs, alcohol, pornography, food, or gambling. If you are tired of putting on a face—of living a lie—then it is time to get real. As hard as it is to be transparent in our culture, each of us needs to open our heart and acknowledge weakness.

It's pride that stands in the way of being real. Ego is the problem.

---

[1] John 16:33 New King James Version

Let's explore this further. Ego, as I have defined it, has two main categories or stages: the Victim and the Controller. These stages are somewhat arbitrarily defined because we can be in both at the same time. But most of the time one of these stages will predominate. The good news is that awakening can happen in either stage. Awakening is the natural outcome of recognizing the ego, seeing its futility, and then choosing a much better alternative.

Stage One: The Victim

In this stage we believe that we are merely innocent victims of everything that is happening to us. This isn't about children who suffer abuse at the hands of others; they are truly innocent. This is about the person who constantly blames others or life events for his or her current situation. The Victim believes that life is a random event and that there is little or no connection between his actions and life consequences. Life's lessons are either misinterpreted to validate the person's dysfunctional belief system or overlooked entirely.

There will always be plenty of evidence to support the victimized mentality. The Victim is naturally drawn to compromised situations and will gravitate toward others of like mind. Such parasitic relationships strengthen and validate the egocentric-driven mind. Yes, misery does love company!

If the Victim over-esteems himself, he will put down others who are succeeding or merely brush off their position to luck. The under-esteemed person will idolize or be jealous of others' success. In either case, "luck" and "bad luck" and "How is life treating you?" make up a regular part of the vocabulary. Feeling sorry for oneself is also common in this stage. The patterns can run deep and begin early in life. Some people will carry victimization right up until the day they die.

From a psychological viewpoint, development of the ego is considered normal. In fact, many educators and parents encourage it in terms of developing self-esteem. In the awakened state, as you will see, esteem is defined in a whole new light.

11

Children quickly incorporate the word "mine" and phrases like "I want that" and, for the Victim personality in particular, "That's not fair!" To the child (and unfortunately for too many adults as well) this crying out for their perceived injustice can easily turn into a habit. The fact that life is not always "fair" is the reality that continues to validate this egocentric attitude. Sibling rivalries and acting out will be common in the extrovert personalities, whereas withdrawing and becoming anti-social will be more common in the introverts. Parents will often feed into the Victim mentality by constantly responding or giving in to the child's inappropriate demands and behaviors.

Lying is another ego trait that begins early as well and will carry right into adulthood with strength if parents do not identify it and deal with it effectively. Part of the thinking process of the young ego is that I can get what I want or do what I want as long as no one sees me or finds out. Yes, this is a normal development phase and can be innocent. If left unchecked, however, it can turn into a more serious issue. Teenagers who have gotten away with lying may be more inclined to experiment with drugs, alcohol, and sexual activity. As this process continues into adulthood, add gambling, infidelity, and financial mismanagement.

Lying and getting away with it is actually fuel for the ego, since the ego believes that I can do what I want, when I want, and how I want. This is a false reality that disregards the laws that govern nature, people, and life. Living in denial enables a person in the Victim stage to believe that no connection exists between his actions and his future. Adults often get caught living a dual life when lying has become a regular habit. This most often leads to a variety of stresses and crisis, to which the Victim mentality will respond, "Oh, why me? Do I deserve this? Life sure isn't fair!"

We can move out of this stage only when we realize and acknowledge that there are consequences for our actions. Many grown-ups never move out of this stage. We are all familiar with the "drama queens and kings" in our lives. These are the people who live in a perpetual state of crisis, yet are constantly blaming everyone and everything for their problems.

The Victim mentality is also true for us when we continue to engage in behavior that is not good for us. Any addiction (be it smoking, food, shopping, sex, etc.) or unhealthy choice (from eating too much saturated fat or sugar to constantly operating in anger mode) has, at its core, pure denial or a separation from reality. We say "I know, I know" when someone warns us about the consequences, yet the words do not have an impact on our hearts or minds. We say foolish things such as, "I'm just going to enjoy my life, and everyone dies anyway." This is irrational justification for destructive behaviors. It is an example of self-victimization, by choosing, whether consciously or not, a compromised life. It is the path of least resistance.

Stage Two: The Controller

In the Controller stage we understand the connection between our choices and their consequences. We perceive that we can get what we want by acting or looking a certain way or by manipulating others. We define who we want to be and find some way to get there. Happiness is whatever we define it, and we're sure that the key to finding it lies within us. Whether we desire money, career, sex, power, or fame, we are sure that if we are smart enough and persistent enough we can get what we want. We can also mirror successful people, write down our goals (and read them 50 times a day), work out, eat a balanced diet, attend seminars, join programs, and read self-improvement books.

An individual with a Victim mentality believes that he or she deserves a better life but has had bad luck. The Controller, however, believes that hard work and natural talents entitle him to the "best" life. This stage is all about exercising our free will in order to benefit ourselves, but without regard as to how it affects others or God.

In this stage, whether we succeed or fail, we are never quite satisfied. Those who succeed only do so on superficial levels. Their happiness depends upon maintaining their carefully designed world. The problem is that the real world is a dynamic one of constantly changing circumstances. You can meet your goals without ever finding happiness. Ironically, if happiness depends only upon our self-defined needs being met and circumstances going our way, we will forever be at the mercy of people and events around us.

Many potentially positive outcomes arise out of living in this stage: having more money, a larger house, a thinner body, etc. The negative results from the "me" mentality are seen all around us: divorce, promiscuity, violence, corruption, disease, stress, even murder. We see children essentially being raised by young daycare workers, employers who view their employees as disposable objects, corporations who dump pollutants into our rivers just to save a few dollars.

We have not done well for ourselves or our world by trying to be in charge, have we? Even when we lead relatively stable, productive lives, highlighted by minutes or hours of happiness, any attempt to reach outside of ourselves, to find meaning in life, to find God, is hindered because we want to define who God is. It is common to hear people say, "I have my own belief in a higher power or God as you call it," or "I don't believe in organized religion but I am a very spiritual person." These are the types of intellectual responses you may hear from someone living in the Controller stage. We want to determine for ourselves what our needs are and how they can best be met. We come up with our own theories on the purpose of life, on our future destiny, and about happiness, in our attempts to quell the unanswered questions.

If we do acknowledge that there is a God, we act like His purpose for existing is to meet our needs and to help us control people, events, and other things in our lives—our own personal genie in a bottle. When things go our way, we give God permission to exist and decide that He is a good God. When events in our lives or in the world don't go as we had hoped, we decide that God is just an abstract concept and, therefore, we really have to take control of the situation ourselves. Thus, even our spirituality is ego-centered. Our form of meditation either focuses on nothing, an abstract concept, or our own desires. Meditation in the Controller stage may help us tune out problems, but it does not heal them. Peace is only temporary, joy is fleeting.

And if a person is honest with himself, he will acknowledge that the sense of "What's the point of all this anyway?" always lurks in the back of his mind.

Stage Two Continued: I Did It My Way

In stage two, the Controller stage, a person often reaches a breaking point because it takes a lot of energy to maintain this false reality. The choices are to slip back heavily into stage one, to move forward defiantly into a stubborn and prideful retreat, or to surrender to God (stage three).

Usually, a crisis or exposure to wrongdoing will bring this decision to a head. If pride and stubbornness prevail, isolation from individuals and former loved ones who stand on principle and refuse to be manipulated will most likely occur. Despite numerous circumstances and opportunities for these individuals to re-evaluate their philosophy of life, behavior patterns, and consequences of poor choices, their ego would rather isolate and hide than to admit wrongs. This ultimately translates into broken relationships, loneliness, and bitterness.

This, in the world's thinking, could be considered a defeated ego. It is far from defeated, however, in the spiritual sense. In fact, a person who gets to this point generally has a hardened heart and will not open the door to his jail even if the key has been left in the lock. These individuals would rather die as a means of laying guilt on those they once loved than to admit guilt. Whether conscious or not, the ego is destructive and has little regard for the welfare of others.

Being awakened from either stage of the ego—the Victim or the Controller—requires a miracle. But the greater miracle is being awakened from the hardened heart of the Controller stage.

Stage Three: The True Believer

Stage three is about surrendering. Not to some religion or

spiritual practice that carries the ego onto an even more convoluted path. Here we surrender to the True Living God, Our Creator and the Creator of all things, Jesus Christ. In Chapter 2, I explain why we must surrender to Jesus Christ.

Finally, we realize that we do not know what is best for us. We tried everything and came up short. Instead of struggling to decide what is most important in life (how we can improve our lives or even how we can best serve others), we surrender our whole being and life to God. If we truly surrender, there will be an actual death of the ego (at least temporarily) as we die to the self and become new creatures.

We turn to God unconditionally. If we are still determined to define God—who He must be and how He must act before we will accept Him—then we are still trying to be God ourselves.

In the True Believer stage, we realize that God is not an abstract concept. He is a real person. He is very specific in His desires and will, His likes and dislikes, and in many of His characteristics much like you or I. Unlike us, He is holy, righteous, and true.

Now awakened, we realize that we cannot manipulate, define, or change God. He exists as He is whether or not we acknowledge His existence. We have three options open to us in response to God: accept Him completely as He is, pretend that He is someone else, or pretend that He doesn't exist at all. We may be frightened to give up control. But to whom are we surrendering? Our Creator, who knows what is best and who wants to bless, protect, and direct our lives.

Finally, we can begin to grow up as we learn to take responsibility for our reactions and responses to others. In the ego stages, we came to believe that every feeling and action was acceptable except guilt. Feeling guilty and making others feel guilty have become the ultimate sins of the modern world. But in the awakened stage we admit guilt, because we are guilty. We accept blame, admit our wrongs, and face our faults head on. This helps us to move beyond the guilt (or the fear of being guilty) to the place where we are able to be forgiven, to be open to change, and to be able to forgive.

Love Redefined

What we call "love" in the ego stages is actually a desire to have the ego gratified, receive validation from others, and avoid acknowledging what needs to be changed within us. It may come in the form of a desire to be loved or to love oneself, but it is ultimately self-centered.

Now awakened, we learn to love others in the way that God loves us. It is easy to love those whom we like, but it requires help from God to love those whom we find annoying, ignorant, unattractive, or uneducated. In the ego stages, love is conditional. In the awakened stage, love is unconditional. That doesn't mean we have to be friends with everyone or agree with their behaviors. But it does require recognition that you and I are simply sinners, saved by grace and grace alone! We no longer chase the mirage called "self-love." It no longer concerns us.

The Bible best sums up what love really is and what it is not: *"Love is patient and kind. Love is not jealous or boastful or proud or rude. Love does not demand its own way. Love is not irritable, and it keeps no record of when it has been wronged. It is never glad about injustices but rejoices whenever the truth wins out. Love never gives up, never loses faith, is always hopeful, and endures through every circumstance."*[2]

If we all had this kind of love, the world would certainly be a better place. Apart from God's help, however, it is impossible to love in this way, because *"God is love"* and *"love comes from God."*[3]

Will I Lose My Sense of Self?

Surrendering to the actual, real God doesn't mean that we lose our personality or that we are absorbed into Him, like a droplet of water into the ocean. God has made each and every one of us unique. No two people in the whole world even have the same

---

[2] 1 Corinthians 13:4-7 New Living Translation
[3] 1 John 4:7-8

fingerprint! God wants us to fulfill the role that He has specifically designed for each of us and live a life that He has planned perfectly for us. Whether we are completely paralyzed or the world's best athlete, in prison or sailing around the world, poor or rich, God has created a special work for each of us. God takes us just as we are! He is the master of repairing broken lives, and He also takes good lives and turns them into great lives. All He requires is a willing vessel that truly gives the Potter all of the clay to work with.

Even after we are awakened, we will slip back into the ego stages from time to time, until we decide that the strife and pain is not worth it and decide to trust God again. There may be areas of our lives or aspects of our personalities that never seem to quite get out of the ego stages. Surrendering to God is a lifelong process. It is difficult, if not impossible, to attain it perfectly here on earth. The good news is that with maturity in our walk with God we can learn to admit our faults quickly and confess our wrongdoings, ask for forgiveness, and then turn fully in the right direction again—all of this under God's amazing grace!

Prayer in the awakened stage is personal communication with God. We bring requests to Him, but also express our desire to submit to His will in all areas of our lives. When we do this, God will change us and put new desires in our hearts.

Meditation involves stillness and quieting of the mind so that we can hear God's voice. It also involves focusing on that which is good, true, and pleasing to God, especially meditating on His Word. Worry can begin to fade and be replaced by faith as we begin to sense and realize God's perfect love for us. We can give our past to God, let Him hold our future, and relax with relief into just living this moment. This doesn't mean that we no longer take action, but as we grow spiritually we begin to recognize more clearly what God calls us to do. When we are God-centered there is no confusion; there is only peace. The mind, body, and spirit are under His direction. What better definition of health can there be?

The process of awakening begins with a simple, sincere desire to change and to know the truth. Do you want to know the truth, no matter the cost? The question is, what is more important to you than knowing the truth, if the truth indeed sets you free? Is social acceptance more important? Is money, or a relationship, or a self-image of intellectualism or political correctness? What could be more important than living in reality and having joy? You have already tried the alternative! Each of us will arrive at the point of surrender in our own way. Sadly, many will never reach that point. Or they may choose, consciously or subconsciously, to go through a great deal of pain before deciding to take that step. A much simpler way is to learn from the experiences of others. We can also learn from taking a good hard look at the experiences of our past, take the lessons to heart, determine to step past the fear, and surrender to reality.

"For I know the plans I have for you," declares the Lord, "plans to prosper you and not to harm you, plans to give you hope and a future.... You will seek me and find me when you seek me with all your heart."[4]

Reflection

Ten questions for small-group discussion or to ask yourself:

1. Can you identify friends or family members clearly stuck in stage one or stage two of the ego? More importantly, can you identify your own egocentric patterns?

2. Have you surrendered to God and become a new creation? If not, what is holding you back?

3. Are there areas in your life in which you are still trying to play God?

4. Do some people in your life really trigger your buttons? What do you think still needs healing in you? Or, what do

---

[4] Jeremiah 29:11, 13

you think God is using this particular person (or persons) in your life for?

5. Are you willing to surrender all your dreams and goals to God? It is good to write a list of your dreams and goals on paper. It is even better to give them all to God and say in your heart, "I want only what You want for my life" or, as Jesus prayed, *"Not my will, but Thy will be done."*[5]

6. Are you willing to admit your wrongs to your loved ones and friends and ask for their forgiveness? Once you understand and receive God's forgiveness, you should be more than willing to forgive others.

7. Are you genuinely interested in the well-being of others and willing to put aside your agenda? Are you loving and kind to your neighbors even if they are unkind to you?

8. Are you willing to examine your words, actions, and thoughts and put them to the test of what God says in His Word to be true and good? Do you find yourself gossiping or talking negatively about others when they are not present?

9. Are you willing to seek the right professional help (*i.e.,* spiritual problems need spiritual solutions)?

10. How do you know when you are actually hearing from or being directed by God? (Here are some clues I've discovered in my life: what I'm hearing doesn't contradict God's written Word; I have a peace about it; most likely it doesn't involve the use of a credit card, more debt, or a high-risk situation.)

Get a notebook to write some commitments you are going to

---

[5] Luke 22:42

make either to face some issues you have been in denial about or to change some habits that are not in your best interest. Review in six months to see your progress!

1.3 The Fallen World

Life is a battle that's won—or lost—daily through our attitude and our choices. Ironically, the choice to surrender is the only choice that assures victory. When we surrender our lives to God, He gives us the victory over every negative thing that comes our way. As soon as we think we are the ones who win victories, we are in big trouble, for as we will learn in Chapter 2, the battles for life, for a good life, are much bigger than us. This is not a battle you or I want to fight alone!

God did not make our instruction manual difficult to interpret or hard to understand when it comes to how to live life. The following simple Bible truths and commands teach us how to live the abundant life. Jesus said the most important commandment in God's law is: *"Love the Lord your God with all your heart and with all your soul and with all your mind and with all your strength."* And the second most important is: *"Love your neighbor as yourself."*[6]

The world is not supportive in helping us to remember these truths. In fact, the temporary ruler of this world, satan, has distorted and confused the simple plan that God has laid out for us to live the abundant life. Jesus calls satan a thief who desires to steal and kill and destroy anything that is good.[7] He is the founder of the egocentric life. Both believers and non-believers can and do become victims to his deceptions and lies, leading to the exact opposite of the abundant life—the miserable life! Living apart from God's commands and truths makes us vulnerable to the wiles of the devil. Living life this way is a difficult road filled with obstacles, hairpin turns, and dangerous cliffs. The Bible is very clear that sin may be fun for a season but in the end leads to destruction.

---

[6] Mark 12:30-31
[7] John 10:10

Myths You Won't Find in the Bible

Satan distorts, deceives, confuses, and lies. Many people have incorrect ideas about what it means to surrender to God.

⇒Myth 1: Honest People Do Not Get Anywhere

It is easy to fall into the trap of looking around at the lives of other people and ask, "What's the point of trying to live an honest life when those who are getting ahead and living comfortably march to the drumbeat 'whatever it takes'?" Actually, the Bible teaches that working hard to achieve one's goals is honorable in and of itself, but the problem runs deeper. Our hearts are never satisfied and we end up messing up in one if not more areas of our lives. Infidelity, addictions, anger, and lying are just some of the fruits of a selfish life that have serious consequences.

Furthermore the Bible says, *"Cast but a glance at riches, and they are gone, for they will surely sprout wings and fly off to the sky like an eagle."*[8] We all know of people who had it all and then lost it all.

And most importantly, *"The blessing of the LORD makes a person rich, and he adds no sorrow with it."*[9]

⇒Myth 2: Money Is the Root of All Evil

Money is not the problem. The problem is our heart. *"No one can serve two masters. Either he will hate the one and love the other; or he will be devoted to the one and despise the other. You cannot serve both God and Money."*[10] Does this mean we are supposed to be poor? Yes, but only in the spiritual meaning of the word—being humble and recognizing our need for God in all areas of our lives.

---

[8] Proverbs 23:5
[9] Proverbs 10:22 New Living Translation
[10] Matthew 6:24

Remember the Bible clearly states, *"For the love of money is at the root of all kinds of evil. And some people, craving money, have wandered from the faith and pierced themselves with many sorrows."*[11] *"But godliness with contentment is great gain. For we brought nothing into this world, and it is certain we can carry nothing out."*[12]

Money is important to people and it should be. You'll find more than a hundred references to money in the Bible, so money is obviously a tool that God uses for His purposes as well.

Getting rich is just one of many temptations and distractions in this world that are illusions of happiness. Part of the awakening process is to realize that you can live in this world and yet not be of this world. God may have blessed you with a great husband or wife, a big house, a nice car, and a fat bank account, and yet your heart and mind can be and should be serving Him alone. One thing is for sure: "No one can serve two masters.... You cannot serve both God and Money."

⇒Myth 3: Only Weak People Need God

This myth is actually true, only weak people do need God. What's left unsaid, however, is that the Bible calls all of us weak. There is no other kind of people. It is only when we die to self and receive the power of the Holy Spirit that we become powerful and have eternal life. *"For you have been born again. Your new life did not come from your earthly parents because the life they gave you will end in death. But this new life will last forever because it comes from the eternal, living word of God. As the prophet says, 'People are like grass that dies away; their beauty fades as quickly as the beauty of wild flowers. The grass withers, and the flowers fall away.'"*[13]

Thus the "strong" people of this world are simply egotistical

---

[11] 1 Timothy 6:10 New Living Translation
[12] 1 Timothy 6:6-7 King James Version
[13] 1 Peter 1:23-24 New Living Translation

delusions. It takes a lot more strength for a person to acknowledge his shortcomings and to ask for forgiveness. Humility or being humble should not be confused with being weak. God uses the weak things of this world to confound the "wise" things of this world.

⇒Myth 4: The Spiritual Life Is Boring

I can personally testify that this is far from the truth. In fact, it is a complete lie. The life of faith is extremely fulfilling and challenging at times, but full of hope, joy, peace, and gratitude when we keep our eyes focused on God.

Put on your sword, O mighty warrior!
You are so glorious, so majestic!
In your majesty, ride out to victory,
defending truth, humility, and justice.
Go forth to perform awe-inspiring deeds!
Your arrows are sharp,
piercing your enemies' hearts.
The nations fall before you,
lying down beneath your feet.
Your throne, O God, endures forever and ever.
Your royal power is expressed in justice.
You love what is right and hate what is wrong.
Therefore God, your God, has anointed you,
pouring out the oil of joy on you
more than on anyone else.[14]

Yes, we are considered royalty when we become God's children. Don't ever be deceived that what the world (the world's philosophies and lusts) has to offer will come close to what God has to offer His children.

The Bible is clear that sin is fun for a season but in the end

---

[14] Psalm 45:3-7 New Living Translation

leads to destruction. I do not want moments of "excitement" in exchange for a lifetime of bitter consequences, and I hope that you don't either. The Lord does give us plenty to be thankful for right here and now, and for those of us who are going to heaven, the eternal rewards cannot even be fathomed. The Bible says, *"No eye has seen, no ear has heard, and no mind has imagined what God has prepared for those who love him."*[15]

If you have become a child of God by accepting Jesus Christ as your Savior, you have entered into eternity with God the moment you made that decision. As the perfect Father, God loves to bless His children and gives us favor, opportunity, and victory over sin. *"Every good and perfect gift is from above, coming down from the Father of the heavenly lights, who does not change like shifting shadows."*[16]

Reflection

Ten questions for small-group discussion or to ask yourself:

1. Does talking about spiritual or religious matters make you uncomfortable? How about Jesus Christ and the cross? If so, where do you think that stems from?

2. Money and how we spend it reveals a lot about our personality and priorities. Are you giving 10 percent of your income back to God? Are you being a good steward of the resources that God has entrusted to you? (Take a look at your checkbook to see if some areas need re-evaluation. This is especially true if you have debt.)

3. What are some of the images and concepts you have about God, heaven, and your role in life? Are there some myths that need to be debunked?

---

[15] 1 Corinthians 2:9 New Living Translation
[16] James 1:17

4. Are there any individuals who are people of faith that you see as good role models for yourself? Remember we are all humans who are prone to make mistakes. It is the people who acknowledge their weakness and seek healing whom I look up to.

5. Have you realized that you cannot earn your way to God or to heaven? Which religions promote this concept either directly or indirectly?

6. Did you know that life here on earth was not meant to be miserable and stressful? Are there still some areas in your life that need to be purged, cleansed, or de-weeded? Does your environment reflect this at all?

7. Are you aware of spiritual warfare? Does the enemy, satan, have a stronghold on any area of your life? Do fears, worries, anxieties, negativity, and doubt grip your life? How about addictions? Anger? Jealousy?

8. Are you content with what you have? If not, begin by counting your blessings one by one. Perspective is everything!

9. Are you honest in everything? Or do you justify "white" lies in your life?

10. Are you absolutely sure that you are on your way to heaven? Why or why not?

Chapter 2, "Thriving Spiritually," will discuss and answer this question.

1.4 My Awakening

When I was born, my family lived in a small town on

Vancouver Island in British Columbia. I remember feeling safe and secure in the love of my parents. Our small corner of the world still had a sense of innocence; our neighbors never locked their doors and everyone knew everyone else by name.

Things began to fall apart when I was five. My father became involved with another woman. I was devastated, as was my mother and older sister, Kym. Two years later when my parents officially separated, my mother, sister, and I moved into a small apartment. Each of us dealt with our pain differently. Kym found her "relief" in her friends, and I turned to excelling in school to maintain my sense of order.

Spiritually and emotionally broken, Mom would drag Kym and me to church every Sunday in her attempt to hold what was left of her and her family together. Kym and I would go reluctantly, with our main motivation being lunch and a root beer float at the A&W restaurant after church. I did not understand the value of church, as all I would see was my mother's pain the rest of the week. I would occasionally hear her crying in her room after a long day at work while I would try to prepare dinner. This broke my heart and made me determined to do all I could to make our home a place of peace and order, and maybe even bring my father back. If church made my mom happy, then I was willing to go.

My sister, however, was not as sensitive to our mother's pain and would skip church fairly regularly. Peace at home became even more out of reach when Kym reached her teens. Her friends would hang out at our house, leaving a mess of cigarette butts, empty beer bottles, and dirty dishes. I earned money on a paper route and occasionally paid my friends to come home with me after school to help me clean up before Mom got home from work. My reward was the smile on her face when she found a clean house waiting for her.

By this time, I had re-established a relationship with my dad. For a brief time I managed to create a sense of relative balance, though I still struggled with inner peace. Then my sister confided to me that she was pregnant and begged me not to tell our parents. Only 15 years old, Kym was confused and lost. By the time she was six months pregnant, she could no longer conceal the truth.

She told my mom, who was shocked. Later, she told my dad. My mom's Catholic upbringing made abortion out of the question, and thankfully so—today my sister's "mistake" is a beautiful young woman, my niece. But at the time, I was overwhelmed by the chaos and moved out to go live with my dad and his new love interest.

Born for Naturopathy

I was a quiet, sensitive child who, because of my own pain, was able to tune into what other people were feeling and the pain that they carried inside. Later, this enabled me to become the type of physician who views an individual as a whole being—mind, body, and spirit—not as a disease condition. Throughout my childhood, I observed the people around me and noticed that some always seemed to have troubles in life and carry pain, while others seemed to be happy-go-lucky. I wanted to understand these differences. Even at a young age I preferred to spend time with adults and observe them. Because of my personality and sensitivity to dysfunction, I decided that I did not want to be like my parents, nor like most of their friends. I quickly moved from the Victim (stage one ego) to the Controller (stage two ego). I wanted order and meaning to my life. I chose to do well in school, hang out with the "good" crowd, and participate in music, sports, and student government. Church was no longer a part of my life.

Although I continued to excel in school, the underlying stress was beginning to catch up with me. My vision began to deteriorate and I developed acne. My father took me to a dermatologist, who prescribed antibiotics (tetracycline). I should have known that the dermatologist could not help me since he had acne himself. After three months, not only did my acne worsen, but I also experienced frequent indigestion. I now know these symptoms were related to a candida (yeast) infection. This was the beginning of my interest in health issues. I became more and more aware of the variety of health issues that people faced. My own grandmothers had chronic health problems. One grandma had cancer and the other diabetes.

As their health deteriorated, I would often ask my parents what good are doctors if they are unable to help.

At the time, one of my father's friends had been studying for years to become a naturopathic physician. Recognizing my interest in health, my dad asked his friend to send me some information. Even though my dad was unable to provide for my emotional and spiritual needs, he loved me and wanted me to do well in life. When I read the brochure on naturopathy, I knew that this was what I wanted to devote my life to. The foundational philosophy made so much sense. The brochure spoke of six principles:

1. First do no harm
2. The healing power of nature
3. Identify and treat the cause
4. Heal the whole person
5. The physician as teacher
6. Prevention is the best cure

Years later, these principles still make a lot of sense. The only major missing point in school was how to address the whole person. Without including God and His healing power of transformation, the whole person cannot be effectively addressed or treated. Nonetheless, God's creations—herbal medicine and food—are powerful medicines that many healing traditions use to bring about improved physical health. My naturopathic training was comprehensive, consisting of conventional medical sciences and the use of diet, exercise, nutrition, herbal medicine, and homeopathy to restore health. I am glad I got this training.

Having this goal in my life at such an early age helped me to stay focused and gave me a sense of purpose. I felt compassion for people who were suffering physically and strongly desired to help them and myself.

In many ways, however, my goals were a distraction from confronting and dealing with some deep pains that I was carrying. It wasn't until I began writing this manuscript several years ago that I uncovered some deep resentment toward my dad. I am happy to report that after a lot of prayer and reconciliation, I am finally free from all of those negative emotions. I believe that those early traumas still affect my sister's decisions to this day. The fact that Kym has not committed to marriage and her tendency to avoid talk about God is evidence to me of this. My sister and I reacted very differently to our painful circumstances and yet we are both compassionate, caring people who care about the welfare of others. I hope and pray that she will also see that the only true healing comes from God and God alone.

Life at the University

Things were going well in my life outside the home. I was elected president of my high school's student council, excelled in music, and had good friends. Life at home, however, was not happy or stable. After several years the relationship between my father and his girlfriend began to fall apart. I often found myself in the middle of their discord and anger. In the process of time, I had actually grown fond of my dad's live-in girlfriend and so the whole process felt like ripping up old wounds. In order to deal with the stress, I would escape to my room and sit in solitude. I soon discovered that I could tune out most of the negative things in my life by focusing on good things. I later realized that I was practicing a form of meditation. In my meditations I included prayers to God, but it was not until I was 21 that I came to know God personally, in the process that I have defined as awakening.

I graduated from high school and began to pursue my goal of becoming a naturopathic physician. Most of the students starting university were experiencing independence for the first time. They spent their freedom on non-stop partying, alcohol, and dorm food. In contrast, I abhorred chaos and the misery it brings. I was attracted to the lifestyle of the seniors who lived in the brand-new university condominiums. Unfortunately, you had to be 21 to live there, and I was only 19. I prayed that God would open the doors for me, and before I knew it I was living with the seniors.

I made prayer and meditation part of my routine while I was at the university. Looking back, I now realize that much of this spiritual discipline was egocentric. I felt that God was supposed to take care of my every need and desire, and if He didn't I needed to pray harder. I knew very little about God, His likes and dislikes, and what He desired for me. Even though I received some physical benefits from my spiritual practices, they were superficial; I knew I was missing out on something deeper.

Each summer I returned to my hometown to work at the paper mill that employed my father and grandfather and earned enough money to cover my tuition. I lived with my father in a two-bedroom apartment. My dad's patterns continued and he began to see yet another woman with three children. She owned a small convenience store close to where we used to live. Apparently her marriage was virtually over when my father met her. After she read my father's palm, they believed that they were soul mates. I was shocked to discover one night that my dad still had not fully cut off his previous relationship. An angry confrontation ended in an emotional and physical wrestling match, after which I stormed out. I pleaded with my grandfather to let me stay with him and he eventually gave in.

My grandpa is a no-nonsense, disciplined, somewhat inflexible man. Under that hard outer core, however, is a soft, loving tenderness. That summer with Grandpa was life-changing for me. I learned to be more ordered and disciplined. Grandpa taught me many skills, including home projects and automobile repairs, which he is still teaching me to this day.

Then I Met Katy

At the end of the summer, I headed back to university to complete my final year of undergraduate work. Until this time, I had been so focused on my goals that I had never allowed myself to have any serious relationships. My Iranian friend and roommate invited me to a Persian concert with him on a night that forever changed my life. Katy (Katayoun in the Farsi language) shook my hand as he introduced us, and it took what seemed like an eternity to break contact with her beautiful brown eyes. I told her of my dreams of becoming a naturopathic physician and eventually opening a wellness center and spa. She was studying economics at the University of Victoria.

Over the next several weeks, as I tried to meditate I found that I could not get Katy out of my mind. Finally, I asked my friend if he could invite her over for dinner the next time she was in town. We started to date and eventually she introduced me to her parents. They were formal with me at first, but I immediately saw how close their family was. My heart longed to be part of a "functional" family. I thought that would meet the emotional needs that my family could not meet.

As the school year ended, I had a dilemma. I needed to earn enough money for medical school in Portland, Oregon, but I dreaded going back to the paper mill and direct dealings with my dysfunctional family. I wanted a new and challenging experience that would help me to grow spiritually and challenge me physically and mentally.

I certainly got what I wanted!

Whatever Was I Thinking?

During the six months since I met Katy, I had virtually abandoned my meditation routine, and my grades had dropped significantly. When I realized how out of balance I was, I quickly got back into my routine and prayed for guidance about my work situation and my relationship. Three days later, one of my roommates enthusiastically told me about his summer job. For the second summer in a row he planned to go door-to-door, selling educational books.

At first I wasn't interested, but his excitement intrigued me. I asked how much he had made the previous summer. "Close to $9,000 American," he replied. That's about what I had earned at the paper mill. I went to my room that evening and meditated and prayed for several hours. I felt excited about this opportunity that would challenge me and probably help me to grow as well. My dad and grandfather were skeptical when I told them what I was planning. They said half seriously, "Don't come running back here for help when you can't afford your tuition." I replied, "Don't worry, I won't!" and took it as a challenge. I spoke with Katy and announced that I honestly didn't know what the future held for our relationship. I told her I would write.

Three days later I was on the road with three other "bookies" in a cramped Honda Civic on our way to Nashville, Tennessee, for training. I had $250 and a determination to do well. After a week of intensive training, I was assigned my territory in Burlington, Ontario, along with three other students. We had a budget of $25 a week to cover room and board. Fortunately, my roommate, who had done this before, found us a place to stay that first night.

As my roommates fell into bed exhausted, I was frightened and having second thoughts about my decision. I sat up late, meditating and praying while everyone else slept. The alarm shattered my sleep at 6:00 a.m. I shivered in a cold shower (part of the inspirational routine), dressed, and was standing in front of the first door at 8:15, thinking that this plan was absolutely crazy. I finally gathered enough courage to knock on the door. No answer. I thought I should move on. I knocked again. An old man swung open the door and shouted, "What do you want!" I started to reply, but he slammed the door in mid-sentence.

I thought, *Oh no, Grandpa and Dad were right. How will I ever face them again? How will I ever pay for school?*

The rest of the week was essentially the same. By the end of the week, I was overcome with fatigue and couldn't hold back the tears any longer. I found a large tree at the corner of someone's front yard, curled up under it, and fell asleep. I woke to the sound of a man's voice saying, "Are you okay, are you okay?" How embarrassing! There I lay in this stranger's yard with my green book bag and grass and twigs dangling from my hair.

"Oh yes, I'm fine. I wanted to take a nap and your tree looked very inviting."

Just as I was ready to walk away, he said, "So, what are you doing out here, anyway?"

"Oh, I'm a student and this is my summer job, selling educational books."

"Would you like me to tell you who on this street has kids?" he asked.

That day I made my presentation to three families. Though I didn't make a sale, at least I went home that evening with a positive attitude. Worry, however, was beginning to settle in, as I hadn't made any sales. How was I going to pay for my tuition? Each week the sales group from the entire area gathered to share success stories and do role-playing. With nothing positive to share, I didn't want to hear about anyone else's successes. Many of the individuals in the group had already made hundreds of dollars and some even thousands of dollars in their first week of selling. Many of them had an unwavering faith that seemed unusual to me. They encouraged me not to give up, and a few said they would pray for me.

I returned to my room that evening praying for guidance. Did I really make the wrong choice coming here? Why then did I feel like I was led to do this? Then I thought, *maybe this is my lesson, to learn humility and admit to my family that I was wrong?* Because I am not a quitter, I pulled myself together and committed to one more week.

By the end of the week, defeated, depressed, and tired, I carried out the routine halfheartedly. No matter how hard I tried to motivate myself, I could not snap out of my funk. Walking down a quiet, lifeless residential street, I finally decided I'd had enough. Strangely, however, I felt drawn to one more house, where there was a light on and a welcome sign on the door. "This is it...my final attempt to sell a set of books," I said to myself.

This Is Too Weird

A woman answered my knock on the door and invited me in. Surprised, I asked, "Don't you want to know what I'm doing?"

"No," she said, "I was praying earlier and I believe you were meant to be here."

This is too weird! I thought.

"Come in and take a seat," she said reassuringly. "Can I get you some tea or coffee?" (Her husband was getting the kids ready for school, which reassured me they were a "normal" family.)

"No, I'm fine," I replied, as I sat on the sofa.

After some light conversation, I was about to give her my book spiel when she said, "Let's talk about why I believe you are here." Startled, I shut my mouth and listened intently.

"God is calling you to an important spiritual path. You are so special to Him, and He loves you and cares for you deeply. He desires to have a personal relationship with you through His Son, Jesus. With your permission I will say some prayers for you, as this road can be challenging."

Though she spoke softly, her words had incredible power that pierced my heart. She gently put her hand on my forehead and began talking in words I could not understand. Suddenly, I felt a gentle wind in the room and a peace unlike anything I had felt before encompassing me. I closed my eyes and perceived a light that kept getting brighter and brighter. Overwhelmed, I fell to my knees and began to sob. Startled, I opened my eyes to see her calm, comforting smile. She asked me if I was okay. "Something strange is happening to me," I said. After explaining it to her, she smiled again and then proceeded to tell me not to worry. "I believe you are experiencing the presence of the Holy Spirit," she said.

I lost all track of time and space and just sat in awe of everything I had just experienced, and then this woman asked me to tell her about my plans for the future. I told her I was going to move to Portland, Oregon, to study naturopathic medicine. She responded with excitement, but at the same time warned me that I would be exposed to many deceptions about healing both in naturopathy and in Oregon in particular. "You don't need to understand everything now," she said, "but remember this moment."

She asked if I was in a serious relationship. I told her that I really loved someone but was unsure of our future. She went on to explain that we must not be intimate until marriage as it was a sin and would have negative consequences. I took what she said seriously. Then she said that whoever I chose to be with must accept my journey and hopefully embrace it.

Before I left she asked me what I was doing in Ontario. I told her about my crazy summer job selling educational books, and she immediately said she would buy a set and proceeded to write a check. Then she asked me to return so that I could attend church with her family. I agreed and left her house still in shock.

I walked a few blocks in a daze and sat down on the curb, feeling overwhelmed. *Was that a dream or did it really happen?* I thought. *It really happened, I can't deny it.* And then I thought, *Oh my God, God is real and He loves me personally!* I had a hard time grasping that mentally, but felt changed in a way that words cannot express as I accepted God into my heart. I knew that my life would never be the same from that moment on. (Now that I've had plenty of years to reflect and understand what it means to be a Christian, I know it's not important to have a 4th of July experience to receive God. I know plenty of solid believers who simply made that decision to receive Christ and then slowly but surely matured in their spiritual walk. No fireworks or mind-boggling experiences.)

That day I presented the books to three other families and every one of them made a purchase. I was stunned and noticed how differently people were reacting to me. My mother had dragged me to church for many years and I believed in God, but never before had I experienced anything like this. That night, my roommates noticed that I was different. I had a glow about me. I told them about my successful sales, but didn't tell them about my life-changing experience. The story just seemed too weird. Before bed, I wrote to Katy that I thought I was truly blessed and that there really was a God. I now realize not only was I baptized by the Holy Spirit but also I had a spiritual anointing upon me—an extra outpouring of the Spirit of God to achieve a specific spiritual purpose.

The following week, I excitedly returned to the woman's house—I was so overwhelmed by the experience that I do not even remember her name. After meeting the rest of her family, we headed off to church. I wasn't sure what to expect, but went with an open mind.

Everyone greeted me warmly, as if they had known me for years. It was definitely different from the church I had grown up in. Just before the service was to begin, I was asked to come to the front to be introduced. The minister put his hand on my back and proclaimed, "This man has been reborn in the Spirit and we all need to celebrate and pray for him today." Everyone stood up and clapped. The minister then asked everyone to be seated and to say a prayer for my protection. As he began the prayer, I felt deeply moved spiritually. As I sat through the service, there were moments when I could not stop the tears from flowing. When they sang a hymn, I would close my eyes and it seemed as if there were hundreds if not thousands of voices singing in perfect harmony. Actually, I believe I was hearing a heavenly choir. The Bible says there's a party in heaven when even one sinner repents and accepts Jesus Christ as his personal Savior.

1.5 No Coincidences

What did the minister mean when he said I was "reborn in the Spirit"? It sounds silly now, but at the time I thought I could turn into an angel, or be forced to become a minister or priest, which didn't appeal to me at all. Determined not to lose control—and become someone, or something, I didn't want to be—I quickly retreated back into the ego stage and focused on the job at hand.

Each week my book sales increased and I was attracting attention from the corporate leaders of the book company. They asked me to share my sales techniques with all of the other sales people. I told them that I wasn't doing anything special, just showing the books. I knew, however, that something had changed ever since that day at the woman's house. People reacted differently to me. When I entered their homes and showed them the books, they would ask me to stay for lunch or dinner. They wanted me to talk to their children. Often, as I left their homes, they would say "God bless you." Some even offered to read Scripture and pray for me. By the end of the summer I had sold close to $30,000 worth of books and won the top First Year Sales award. I earned $12,000, more than enough to pay for my first year of medical school. (When I showed off my check to my grandfather and dad, they were at a loss for words, but I could tell they were proud of me.)

Meanwhile, I continued to write to Katy and felt like we were developing a spiritual connection. I realized she was the woman I wanted to share the rest of my life with. When I flew back to Vancouver, the first thing I did was to buy Katy a promise ring. I told her I wanted to marry her and the promise ring symbolized my commitment to her. With tears in her eyes, she put the ring on her finger.

My first day of medical school was only four days away. Katy agreed to drive with me to Oregon to help me get settled. We arrived on Friday afternoon; school started on Monday. Katy gave me a hard time about not finding a place to live before this. I told her not to worry and to trust in God, but she seemed skeptical. Even though I had made good money, I still needed to budget for living expenses and food. I fully believed that God was going to provide for all of my needs. To Katy, however, it looked like I had gone off the deep end.

We first checked the college bulletin boards to see if there were any postings. I called on a few places listed, but they had already been taken. We drove down a street near the college and I spotted a nursing school. I wondered if they had some residency space available at a reasonable price. I walked into the reception area and explained my situation to the receptionist at the front desk. She said the dorms were only for nursing students, and they were full.

Just as I was turning to leave, I overheard a staff member on the phone saying, "If your daughter wants to look after the house, she has to let the woman know today." As soon as she hung up, I asked her about her conversation. She explained that a nurse and her husband were looking for someone to housesit and care for their cats while they were working out of state. I told her my situation and she gave me their phone number. Fifteen minutes later, I was unpacking my car and meeting the cats. All I had to pay for were the utilities. I smiled at Katy as she looked at me in amazement. I felt blessed and thanked God for watching over me.

God Was Indeed Changing Me

The school year flew by. I could not stop thinking about what had happened in Ontario. Amazingly, the man who owned the house I was living in had also had a life-changing experience in which he came to know God. We talked at length about our experiences. Seeing my curiosity to know more about God, he gave me my first Bible. Like an infant hungry for milk, I thirsted for more knowledge about God and read the Bible every night.

In Ontario I was concerned that I would be changed into someone else. I soon realized that God was indeed changing me, and for the better. I felt the deepest gratitude that God was interested in me and wanted a personal relationship—an active, living relationship. I also came to understand that God is always there for me and that He never changes. If I ever felt distant from Him, it was I who had gone astray. God would not reject me, now that I had accepted Him as God. Most importantly, I realized that this life wasn't about me at all. I lived in order to serve Him, and He would be responsible for anything that I accomplished. All of my shortcomings and mistakes I could surrender to Him as well! As His child, I would receive blessing upon blessing. My duty and privilege is to trust and obey Him, always putting Him first in my life.

Meanwhile, Katy was living in Vancouver and visiting me once a month. Partly because of my fear of how she would react, I didn't expand on my deep hunger for God's Word and my relationship with Him. I was living a double life and not always honest with her or with God, which is a recipe for disaster. We were in love and I didn't want her to think that I had become some sort of religious fanatic.

I soon found a church close to my home. A few months later, when I learned about water baptism, I felt called to be baptized. Afterward, an older woman in the church came up to me and handed me a note. It said that she saw angels around me and a bright light over my head. She said that there are celebrations in heaven when someone commits his life to God, and that He was pleased with my commitment. The lady then told me that God would walk with me through my entire life but that, if I ever struggled, I should reflect back on this moment. Her message was strikingly similar to that of the woman in Ontario.

I felt a profound peace in my heart and truly longed to serve God. But even though I wanted to share my experience with others, I felt unable to express what God was doing in my life because of my fear of rejection. At school, they were teaching us that spirituality plays an important role in health and disease. As I began to work with more patients, I became convinced that many health problems stemmed directly from the absence of a prayer life, lack of faith, and disharmony between how God wants us to live and how we actually do live. I wanted to tell these patients about God's amazing love for them, but because of my own weakness and my profession's teachings, I kept quiet. I was becoming a secret service Christian in my attempt to be open-minded and well-rounded.

Sick in Medical School

By the second year of medical school, I was starting to feel the stress of living on a shoestring. I worked occasional odd jobs just to put food on the table. With my heavy class load and the financial strain, my immune system began to falter. Our dissection lab used formaldehyde to preserve the bodies, and my system did not tolerate the fumes well. I soon developed constant fatigue and a chronic sore throat, along with multiple chemical and food sensitivities that no one at the clinic could seem to help me with. How ironic—I came to medical school to learn about health but had become sick.

I prayed and meditated but discovered no answers. In the clinic they told me to follow a vegetarian diet; I only became weaker. They put me on vitamins, herbs, and homeopathic remedies, which only provided temporary relief at best. I did hydrotherapy, colonics, and juice fasts, which offered short-term boosts in energy. If I ate only steamed vegetables, fish, brown rice, and chicken, I could function. Any other foods made my mind foggy and my throat inflamed. When the school installed new carpets, the chemicals caused a constant burning in my eyes and throat.

Frustrated by the conflicting and ineffective advice I received from various clinic practitioners, I decided I had to figure out what to do on my own. My faith in God had not wavered. Remembering a phrase from the Bible, "Physician, heal thyself," I began to meditate on and pay attention to what was happening within my body. I soon became aware of my shallow breathing patterns. I learned that I could feel better simply by doing five minutes of deep breathing. Also, I became aware that I wasn't chewing my food thoroughly—too much eating on the run, not taking the time to enjoy a meal. I discovered that whenever I ate something sweet, including fruit, my sore throat worsened. I finally realized that I must have been harboring some sort of organism that thrived on sugar.

One day in our lab class we were to bring in a stool sample to analyze under the microscope. When I looked at my sample, my suspicions were confirmed. I identified yeast-like spores that I suspected were candida. I had learned a bit about this in one of our classes. Feeling a little embarrassed by the discovery of an organism in my stool, I did not tell anyone. I went straight to the college library and read everything I could find. I found that I had symptoms of adrenal fatigue and candida, which included fatigue, recurrent sore throat, food and environmental sensitivities, and brain fog. For the candida, the books recommended a list of nutrients and herbs including caprylic acid, Pau D'arco, and garlic. To my amazement, that same afternoon a nutritional supplement company set up a table at the college to display some products. I found a supplement that contained many of the ingredients I had just read about, along with some unfamiliar herbs. I bought the product and eagerly ran to the fountain and swallowed four pills. Not long after taking the pills, I broke into a cold sweat, my glasses steamed up, and I almost fainted. I realized that I might be having a die-off reaction, caused when the dying yeast releases toxins. I was excited that I had finally found the answer, but realized that I needed to continue at a slower pace.

As I took the product daily, avoided sugars, and practiced deep breathing, my symptoms steadily improved. Most of my food and environmental sensitivities also improved, though I noticed a slight setback when I ate too much wheat, sugar, or dairy products. Symptoms also worsened if I did not get enough sleep or experienced extra stress, such as when I had to study for an exam. After diligently following my self-made program for six weeks, I was virtually symptom-free. Eventually I had the mercury amalgams removed from my teeth. This seemed to help my immune system, although not dramatically as some people experience. I felt totally empowered by my discoveries and wanted to help others become empowered through directing their own healing processes. I had suffered with this illness for almost two years, but had learned so much from it, personally and professionally. The experience helped me to understand my own body much better and gave me the compassion I would need to be a good practitioner. I began to understand that difficult experiences can ultimately be a blessing.

Over that year, I knew Katy was frustrated in Vancouver. She had just graduated with a degree in economics and was working in a clothing store designing window displays. She had never quite found her calling in life and I wanted to help. I knew that she was very creative and loved fashion, so I arranged an interview for her with a fashion school in Portland. I didn't tell her in advance, but surprised her when she came to visit. An hour after dropping her off for her interview and tour at the school, she came out the door smiling. "This is what I have always wanted to do," she said. "I just didn't know it!" I thanked God for helping me to lead her to this and felt that He wanted us to be together.

God's Sign on a Winding Road

Katy excelled in school and became resident manager at her dorm. I brought her to my church and began to tell her more about what had been happening to me. This was all new to her and hard for her to understand, but she supported me anyway. When she accompanied me to church, however, some of the people acted distant and almost unfriendly toward Katy, and their attitude toward me seemed to change as well. Although they may have been concerned that she would hamper my relationship with God because she was not a believer, they didn't express it in an appropriate or loving way. Rather than seeking God's will in this situation, I simply stopped attending church, though I continued to study on my own. I didn't want anything or anyone to interfere with my relationship with Katy. I didn't realize the importance of connecting regularly with people who shared my beliefs and that this was God's desire as well.

With each passing day, despite my own shortcomings, God was still lovingly watching over me and gently calling me back to a deeper walk with Him.

During my third year in school, Katy and I began talking seriously about marriage. Katy found the differences between our families stressful. One rainy night, while we were driving to pick up a video, she said that perhaps we should "forget the whole marriage thing." I tried to reason with her, but she was emotional, frustrated, and depressed. Suddenly, a speeding car appeared around a curve on the winding road and collided with us, ramming Katy's door. I saw the entire accident as if in slow motion and grabbed Katy's head just as the impact jolted us across the street. By the grace of God, the only injury was my minor cut and bruised hand, though we were both shaken up.

We climbed out of the car through my door, and Katy began apologizing. Confused, I asked why she was apologizing to me. She said, "I'll tell you later." The ambulance and police soon arrived, and after the paramedic determined that we were fine, Katy and I walked to her place. As we walked, her thoughts came spilling out. She said that while we were driving, she had been thinking that she didn't want to go through the stress anymore. Though she loved me, our backgrounds were too different. *Unless I have some sort of sign from God,* she thought, *I don't want to get married.* Moments later, we narrowly missed serious injury, perhaps even death. In that instant, Katy realized how fragile our lives are, and that everything she had been worrying about was small and irrelevant. A feeling of peace came over her, and then she said that she knew I was the man she should marry. Despite our aches and pains from the accident, we started laughing and crying and reaffirming our love for each other.

Not long after, I asked Katy's parents if I could marry their daughter. Both were very accepting and loving, but wanted me to finish school first. I agreed that it was a wise decision, given the heavy course load and clinic schedule I still had ahead of me.

My Own Mish-Mash Spirituality

During those last couple of years I was so busy at school that I stopped praying as frequently and didn't read the Bible at night. In addition to attending naturopathic college, I had decided to get a master's degree in Oriental medicine, which included the study of acupuncture and Chinese herbs. I began to learn about Taoism and Buddhism, and I practiced Tai Chi and Qigong and found significant health benefits from them.

Once again, in my attempt to avoid being narrow-minded, I began to embrace Eastern philosophies. After a while, I didn't know what I believed anymore and became thoroughly confused. I started to create a new spirituality called mish-mash. People even responded to my mish-mash and liked what I was saying. A little meditation, a little deep breathing, a few chants, a new soul, an old soul, trust your heart and feelings, and, oh yeah, let's not forget about God. Even though I felt intellectually good about how I was able to incorporate multiple beliefs into a new, bigger picture, my heart began to grow emptier and emptier. I wanted to develop my relationship with God and that was blatantly missing in these Eastern "religions." Even when they mentioned God, it was not the one I had come to know. I kept these thoughts to myself.

As graduation approached, I had many sources of stress: financial concerns, wedding preparations, my all-important board exams, and decisions related to starting my practice. When I returned to Vancouver for the wedding, I was nervous about the first meeting between our families. They came from different worlds and had different life philosophies. I was having a hard time keeping everything in the proper perspective.

Unfortunately, my diet was also a stress on my body. Since I arrived in Vancouver, I had been eating all the foods to which I was sensitive. My old symptoms flared up. The night before the wedding I went out with friends and popped a couple of garlic pills to help my sore throat. We were standing in line at the movie theater when I suddenly felt weak and started to faint. I leaned on my friend who walked me to a restaurant to sit down. I was perspiring heavily and knew from previous experience that I was having another candida die-off reaction. That night, as I meditated, I realized that I was worrying about things over which I had no control. I could only do my part at the wedding and leave the rest to God. That settled, I slept well.

The wedding was beautiful; my dad actually showed up in a tux! Between the parties and the honeymoon, we were on cloud nine. Unfortunately, you can't continue to live above your problems. Back in Portland after a whirlwind of festivities, reality struck. We had very little money and didn't know yet if I had passed my exams. Deep inside, I had an assurance that everything was going to work out; nonetheless, we both were stressed. A week later, the envelope from the college board arrived. My heart raced as I ripped it open. I had passed all the exams and could start my practice! Now, the hard work would really begin. I had to build a private practice and earn a living.

After a few months of doing all I could to find new patients, I was barely earning enough to pay our rent. Fortunately, I received an opportunity to work as a physician's consultant for the same nutritional supplement company that made the first candida medication I had used. Working with the doctors who owned the company and researching their products increased my knowledge of nutrition tremendously. For many hours each week, I was speaking with doctors around the country, answering their questions and discussing their patients' cases. I taught at seminars and was in frequent contact with the people who were on the forefront of research in natural medicine. At the same time, my practice took off. Within six months, I had a busy practice and a job I enjoyed.

Growing Discontent Despite Success

Everything, it seemed, was going well. Over time, my practice became very successful. I had many patients and enjoyed excellent relationships with them. I had daily opportunities to treat chronic illnesses and to use my background in naturopathic and Chinese medicine to make a real difference in people's lives. I also joined with others to form a ten-practitioner clinic, where I had a leadership role. My daughter, Tatiana, was born, and her presence in our lives was a blessing that we both enjoyed. Katy and I had wonderful friends and our lives were full. We were comfortable in Portland.

Despite this, my spiritual life was not satisfying. My main spiritual input came from my professional duties, from Eastern spiritual practices, and from interacting with practitioners who also made their own homemade concoction of spirituality. I longed for a closer relationship with God and in-depth relationships with other people who knew Him. At one point, out of my desire to have more spirituality and to find something that would perhaps appeal more to Katy, we attended a New Age church that her friend had suggested. The atmosphere was cozy and the people were genuinely warm. But as time went on, I realized that the messages being taught usually did not match up with the Bible. The messages were what people wanted to hear. At the core was a self-made religion that tried to appeal to everyone. I sensed that "God" was an abstract concept to them, a wonderful idea, and not an actual person with whom they could communicate. I found little value in teachings that weren't based completely on the truth.

The God whom I knew was the same one who created galaxies, atoms, flowers, waterfalls, and thunder. More than that, He knew my every thought, and I could walk and talk with Him throughout my day. He was real, powerful, and—the most mind-boggling of all—He was a loving God. He loved me to an extent that was almost unimaginable, and much more than I, or anyone else, deserved. He deserved to be worshiped wholeheartedly. All this was missing at the New Age church we were visiting.

I wanted so much to share these things with Katy and our

friends, but once again I did not have the courage. My fear of rejection overruled. In my practice and at my workplace as well, I longed to tell people about what had truly brought me health and peace. I could see that the medical information I gave my patients was helpful and the treatments were effective, but I was holding back something crucial. Although the physical relief they felt was important to me, I knew their lives could be much richer and so much more joyful. I could offer them true healing on physical, mental, emotional, and spiritual levels. God began to put a desire in my heart to share more with all of the people in my life about the true healing power of God. More than that, He had put a burning desire in my own heart to draw close to Him once again.

To outsiders, my life seemed successful in every way. I was good at putting on a face, but I sensed that God wanted me to make some major changes. When I realized that I was cheating my patients by not giving them the most positive, life-changing information, my practice slowly became less fulfilling. My involvement at the clinic, which had once been so exciting, was becoming burdensome. My personal growth felt at a standstill. I desired to grow spiritually in my life and with Katy, but I did not know how to accomplish it. I knew our present environment would have to change.

God's Timing Is Perfect

During prayer, I continued to sense that God wanted us to move, but I was reluctant. I constantly argued with myself, seeking to rationalize why I should remain living where I was. How could I leave such a successful practice and abandon my relationship with hundreds of patients? How could I stop working with my present employer? It was exciting, valuable work that offered many opportunities for me to teach and to keep on learning. I felt that if I left, things would fall apart. I sensed that change needed to occur if Katy and I were to grow and even survive in our marriage, yet I felt trapped. The longer I stayed, the heavier my discontent weighed on me. My thinking was very limited, confined to what I thought I could make happen through my own efforts.

A series of events then unfolded, clearly orchestrated by God.

1.6 Holy Fire

One freezing January night, an ice storm hit Portland. In the morning, I awakened to the insistent ringing of our phone. It was one of my patients. Her voice was urgent. "Have you seen the news?"

Snug in my bed, I calmly replied, "No."

"Your clinic is on fire!"

I knew immediately that God was making the changes I had failed to initiate. I calmly went back to sleep knowing that I could not travel on the icy roads and that the situation was beyond my control.

The next day, when the streets were passable, I made my way to the clinic. The damage was significant enough that we could no longer practice in the building. The entire clinic had sustained smoke damage, but surprisingly our individual property was spared for the most part. We soon discovered that it would take approximately three months to repair the clinic. We called a meeting to discuss strategies for finding a new location. I spent time in prayer, asking for courage, and announced to the group that I would not be joining them in the move. As I spoke, it was as if an enormous burden was lifted off my chest. I soon found my own place and my practice was back in full operation within a few weeks. I signed a yearlong lease, knowing that the move was only temporary, and that God wanted me to continue making plans to leave the state.

God's Plan or Ours?

The year flew by. Katy and I continued to investigate possibilities, and I continued to pray about them. Katy expressed a desire to expand her career in fashion. When she mentioned

California, I ran with the idea. I had ulterior motives to leave Portland, which once again I failed to share with her. Almost immediately, doors began opening. I found someone who would take over my practice and some interested buyers for our house. I asked the owner of the nutritional supplement company if he needed anyone to represent the company in California. As I expected, he replied that they had a long-term contract with their sales manager for the entire region, who had represented them for many years. Two months later, much to the surprise of all of us, she put in her resignation. With the opportunity at hand, my wife was now seeing, along with me, that California was the place we ought to be.

We made the move, bought a BMW convertible (part of God's plan I was sure!), and we were off to a fresh start with the California dream and spiritual renewal. I immediately found a church that centered on the Word of God, where people would challenge me to grow spiritually, and where I could worship with others who loved God. Katy was visiting her parents at the time, so I went alone the first time. As soon as the worship songs started, I began to weep uncontrollably. I felt I was back home! My heart and soul were being nourished, and the people had the same intimate connection with God that I once had. The next week, I brought Katy and Tatiana. I wanted to establish right at the outset in this new location that our family would center our lives on God. I felt our lives were back in order, a fresh start.

Everything Fell Apart

But the transition did not go as I had hoped or planned. The sale of our house in Oregon, which we thought was a done deal, fell through. Katy did not embrace the new church that I felt so good about. I thought she would jump in with me to a deeper level of commitment to God. I was wrong. Instead of strengthening our relationship, we were becoming more divided. I felt unsupported and frustrated, and I know Katy did as well. In addition, financial troubles began to mount. I had set out to California to straighten things out. I felt God had led me here, and yet things had become worse than ever! What was happening?

I began to bury myself in my work and developed new friendships with people who could relate to me. Katy would reluctantly attend church at times but felt like everything was being pushed down her throat. I didn't want her to feel this way, so I stopped asking her to come to church and stopped talking to her about God.

While traveling for my work I met a health care practitioner with whom I had a lot in common. I asked her to pray for Katy and me, and she asked me to pray for many problems in her life. She had recently gone through a separation with a man she was totally in love with. She believed that witchcraft was used to break them up, and she looked to my prayers to help restore her life and their relationship. This concept of witchcraft, along with satanic warfare, was foreign to me. My spiritual ego moved me into the savior role, and I began to pray with her daily. This woman intrigued me. She appeared to have a lot of faith, claimed to be psychic, knew a lot about natural medicine, and desired to help me to reconnect to Katy.

It wasn't working. Katy grew more resentful when I would pray with this woman and wanted nothing to do with her. Our relationship was purely platonic and yet it was causing distress between Katy and me. I could not understand why God was allowing this to happen. Not only was my relationship with Katy not getting better and our financial situation crumbling, but the company I had been working for the past eight years was being sold. Katy's insecurities began to mount. Despite all of this, I put my faith in God and trusted that He would see us through this mess and make us stronger in the process.

One day I met for lunch with my newfound prayer partner. While I was sharing with her about our move from Oregon, a large man with tattoos and biker gear approached our table. He said that he had overheard I was from Oregon. I smiled and nodded. He went on to say that he had just returned from riding his motorcycle up to Oregon and had really enjoyed it. I made a polite reply. He continued to stand over our table, and I sensed that he wanted to say something.

"So what brings you over here?" he finally asked. I replied that I was representing a physician's line of botanical and nutritional supplements, and was hoping to open a health spa. He stood there looking at me; the silence was awkward.

"So what brings you over here?" I said finally.

He shrugged and said, "I live in this area." Suddenly, a look of confidence came over him and he said, "Do you mind if I say a prayer over you?"

His words startled me, but I gave him permission. Standing in the middle of the restaurant with people watching, he put his hands over me and prayed, "Dear Lord, I know You have great plans for this child of Yours. Shoot him out like a rocket into this new millennium to bring truth and light to all those around him."

As he continued to pray, a familiar feeling came over me. The room began to light up with such intensity that I felt taken back to that experience in Ontario so many years ago.

I realized then, and especially in the months to follow, that God was using the storms in my life to build my character and my trust in Him, to learn spiritual discernment, and most importantly to build courage and boldness. Nothing in life was more important than God, and there was no excuse for my remaining silent about Him.

God had much bigger plans for me than I had envisioned for myself. My life's work would be to minister to others using everything that God had given me: my medical training, my experience with my patients, and all that I had learned about Him, seamlessly woven together. I could care for others in a truly holistic way, helping them to bring mind, body, and spirit under the direction of God, and I would be learning right alongside them.

The stress and challenges, however, did not end here. A month later I lost my younger half-brother in a tragic car accident. On top of it all, our finances had gotten even worse. I kept on leaning on God for understanding, but I was feeling overwhelmed and depressed. My pride kept me from reaching out to others in a way that I needed to, but I still sensed God was in control and I trusted Him.

Meanwhile, I kept on praying with this other woman and Katy and I drifted further apart. My mom wanted to come to California to stay with us and go to a Marian conference (a Catholic gathering to honor Mary). In her desperation, Katy opened up to my mom about what was happening between us and told her about the woman I prayed with. During the conference, I brought the woman to meet Mom, thinking that she would recognize that Katy was overreacting. The woman encouraged my mom to join her at a prayer meeting. Later, Mom confronted me. She said the woman was pushy and aggressive and coming between Katy and me. Although I argued a little, Mom was right. I asked God for forgiveness, apologized to Katy and asked her to forgive me, and cut off the "relationship" with the woman.

Not long after this, Katy received Jesus Christ as her Savior! This was a reality that made all of our turmoil seem worthwhile to me. I was amazed that in spite of my foolish choices, God opened up Katy's heart to receive Him.

The Miraculous Continues

Soon after that, we received a phone call from our realtor. She said there was a home in a good neighborhood that we might like—a three-bedroom, two-bath, double-garage, two-story condo in a gated community.

That evening we all went to see it and loved it, including my three-year-old daughter. We signed the paperwork to buy it!

The next day I called the mortgage broker I had been working with and told him what I had done. He laughed and said, "You can't buy that with the debt to income ratio you have!"

I was devastated and my wife extremely discouraged. I thought we could ask for help from our parents, but Katy emphatically requested that we not ask for help from anyone. We had done that before and she did not want that kind of obligation again. I agreed.

The next day, the mortgage broker called and asked why the condo I wanted to buy was priced so low for its size and location.

He said for that neighborhood it should be selling for a lot more. He asked me to check if there was something wrong with it and to get an appraisal. Sure enough, the appraisal came in $50,000 higher than the asking price, and because the house had so much equity already built in, the mortgage broker informed me that we would qualify! I couldn't believe it and neither could Katy.

I was on cloud nine that week and on my knees thanking God for His amazing grace and provision, but a call from the seller nearly ruined everything. He said that his wife, who was leaving him and his daughter, wanted more money for the place. I argued that he already signed a contract, but he assured me that he could get out of it. Once again I was discouraged but put my trust in the Lord. After a lot of prayer, I received a call from the seller who said he'd accept a deal if we would add $5,000 to the offer. Done!

That week we also found out that Katy was pregnant with our second child. God definitely loves to shower His children with blessings. We were thrilled!

The Truth Sets Us Free—Even If it's Painful!

Life was much better in our new home. The neighbors were friendly, there were lots of kids for Tatiana to play with, and there was a pool. The only negative part was that the bills continued to build up and the credit interest was killing us. Each week as I would balance the checkbook, the numbers were not adding up. I kept telling my wife that things would get better, but they didn't.

One day while I was sitting by the pool, one of our neighbors, who I had not met yet, came and sat beside me. After some light conversation, we got into some deep personal issues. He and I connected on many levels as he was also involved in nutrition and had two kids. I opened up to him about our serious debt problem and that I had been trying to protect my wife from how bad it really was. "Hey brother," he said, "just tell the truth to your wife and you will hit rock bottom. But hey, then there will be only one way to go—back up."

I took his advice to heart and shared with my wife just how bad our financial state was. She broke down crying and yelling at me—this went below rock bottom. Still, just telling her the truth lifted a burden that I had been carrying for quite some time.

The next day I shared our situation with the pastor of our church and he offered some good counsel. He said he had seen this scenario many times and had seen people handle it in a number of ways, both good and bad. He encouraged me to avoid bankruptcy at all costs. He recommended trying to work out a payment plan with my creditors first, and God would honor and strengthen us for paying back the debt we owed. It wouldn't be easy, he said, but the rewards for doing things the right way would pay off. He told me about someone who, after several years, had paid off all of his debt and whose life was restored.

I made up my mind that day that I wanted to handle this in a way that would please God. The next day I went to see a debt counselor who advised that bankruptcy was probably my best option. He told me we should sell everything and rent an apartment. His advice did not sit well with me, so I continued to seek help from other sources while praying for guidance. I came across another debt agency that said they could legally help me settle with my creditors for a reduced amount over a three-year period. They would also make sure that we would not be bothered by creditor phone calls. After much prayer and consideration, we decided this would be our best option and had God's peace about the matter.

As I moved out of denial and began to face our problems head on with God's help, our life continued to get better and better. Katy and I grew closer again, and we were excited about our son who was soon to arrive. Things were still a little stressful with the nutritional company that I consulted for because there were so many changes occurring within management. Regardless, I stayed as focused as I could and trusted God for the outcome.

A few months later we went to a convention in Arizona and my old boss asked how everything was going in California. I told him we were doing well but the instability in our new company was making me uneasy. He then asked if we had considered moving back to Oregon so that I could work at the home office again. He was still working with the company and said they could definitely use my support there.

Katy and I looked at each other—the thought sounded pretty good. The following week we thought and prayed about it and came to the conclusion it would be the right move.

Trouble in Katy's Family

Katy's parents made regular visits to California and, with a little prodding, would usually attend church with us. Being Iranian, they were exposed to Islam in their childhood but did not practice any formal religion. Both were American-educated, smart, and successful. Katy's dad was a proud, self-made man dedicated to the success of his family and generous both financially and philosophically in his advice. He told me that a book by Ayn Rand, *Atlas Shrugged,* had helped shape his philosophy of life. From my limited understanding of the subject, it is a book based on existentialism. Existentialism's main concept, derived from Kierkegaard's teachings, is that man is not part of an ordered metaphysical scheme, but that individuals must create their own beings, each in his own specific situation and environment. It is basically each man for himself. As the Bible states, there is nothing new under the sun—simply another version of the egocentric life, which is appealing to most people.

My faith in God irritated and confused Katy's dad. He felt that educated people were supposed to know better than to believe in God and religion. When we had some private time together, sometimes we'd discuss spiritual things, and although he put up a wall that I was not to climb over, he seemed intrigued by my unwavering faith. Every time he came to church with us I considered it a miracle and prayed that God would open his eyes to see the truth.

Well, the Word of God is powerful, and when people hear it they are often convicted of sin and either want to run from God or are drawn to His love. God gently knocks on the door of their hearts and says, "If you invite Me in, I will come in and renew your life." God never forces Himself on anyone. Each time that God gives someone an opportunity to turn from his sin and receive Him, if God is rejected the invitation may become harder to hear. It becomes a matter of man's pride, and the Bible says, *"God sets himself against the proud, but he shows favor to the humble,"*[17] and, *"Pride goes before destruction, and haughtiness before a fall."*[18]

Unfortunately, my father-in-law rejected God, elevated pride...and eventually fell hard. Shortly after the birth of our son, Katy's parents became divided and eventually divorced. This family, whose stability I once found so attractive, descended into complete destruction. The foundational philosophy of my father-in-law was flawed and crumbled once put to the test. The Bible teaches us that the truth truly sets one free, but it can also divide families.

"Don't imagine that I came to bring peace to the earth! No, I came to bring a sword. I have come to set a man against his father, and a daughter against her mother, and a daughter-in-law against her mother-in-law. Your enemies will be right in your own household! If you love your father or mother more than you love me, you are not worthy of being mine, or if you love your son or daughter more than me, you are not worthy of being mine. If you refuse to take up your cross and follow me, you are not worthy of being mine. If you cling to your life, you will lose it; but if you give it up for me, you will find it."[19]

It may be hard to understand why God would do this, but we're reminded that life is serious, and the consequences of sin are dead serious.

In the midst of the beginning of this huge family division, Katy and I had our wonderful son, Alexander. What should have been a peaceful, enjoyable time for my wife turned into a nightmare.

---

[17] James 4:6 New Living Translation
[18] Proverbs 16:18 New Living Translation
[19] Matthew 10:34-39 New Living Translation

More Messes and Miracles

Not long after this stress we sold our condo at a significant profit and paid off about half of our credit card debt. This was clearly God's provision and blessing for us seeking to correct our mistakes in a way that would please Him. We arranged to rent from the buyer for four months so that we could make a smooth transition back to Oregon. I told Katy that while I was in Oregon at a national sales meeting for the nutritional company, I would begin looking for a place to live. Returning to my hotel room one evening, as I was reading Scripture and praying I heard in my mind, "Go buy a house."

"What?" I said.

"Go buy a house!"

I told God that's crazy! How do you buy a house without any credit? But in obedience to what I heard, I called a realtor. After all, I remembered what God had done for us in California. The next day, the realtor came to show me around. I called up my friend Inez who always had a good sense for homes and what my wife would like.

After a few discouraging home viewings and a reality check about prices, Inez encouraged the realtor to drive down a street in a brand-new neighborhood with beautiful big homes. As soon as we walked in the first house, we looked at each other and nodded—this is what Katy would like. Amazingly, the price was only slightly higher than what I had suggested to the realtor.

I called Katy on my cell phone and within minutes I was signing papers to buy a lot for our brand-new house. All I had left from the sale of the condo was $5,000 (after paying down debts). It was the exact amount needed to hold the property on which the house was to be constructed. I got so excited in the moment that I almost forgot that I did not even have a loan approved yet. I had 60 days to get the loan approved, and then they would begin building. In the back of my mind—and front and center in Katy's—I also had only 60 days in which to get our $5,000 back, just in case we were not approved. After all, God may want me to buy a house, but did we really deserve something this nice after the credit mess we created? No, but God's grace and mercy are truly awesome!

Reality struck when I called a lender and he said, "Come back in 10 years, your credit is like broken glass." I thanked him and called another lender. He didn't offer much hope but said he'll give it a shot. That was good enough and I sent him all of our paperwork.

Week after week I'd call to see how things were progressing, and each week I'd hear the same refrain: "Call me back next week." He kept reminding me, "It's a stretch and I'm pulling out all the tricks in my bag." That did not give me a whole lot of confidence.

One day, I was looking at the calendar and I realized that the 60 days had just passed. *O Lord, we cannot afford to lose that $5,000! My wife is going to kill me.* I pulled out the contract and, sure enough, there would be no refund after 60 days. Katy was furious. I told her it was still possible we'd get the financing, but she didn't want to hear that. Another week went by and still no progress. I was mad at myself that I did not pay more attention to the deadline and was getting angry with the lender for not communicating through the process.

I was working when the builder called. Expecting to be scolded for not getting my finance papers in yet, I was surprised when the gentleman said, "What color do you want the shingles?"

"You haven't started building yet, have you?"

Yes, he had! After all, he said, I was a doctor. He never suspected a doctor could have trouble getting a loan.

With that little boost to my ego, I didn't know what to say, so I told him I'd talk it over with my wife and call him back. When I told Katy, she got even madder at me. I explained that we would not be held accountable for any more expenses if we did not get a loan because the builder took his own risk assuming that I would get approved. Over the next three weeks, Katy had a heyday picking out kitchen cabinets, Berber carpet, extra windows, and a few special build-ins. It became kind of a joke—she said that whoever gets this house is going to really enjoy it!

Meanwhile, the lender finally got back to me and said, "Hey buddy, it really doesn't look like I can make this happen!" Here came another of those moments that forced me to stop living in denial and face the problem head on. I had to call the builder and be honest with him. Not fun!

I called him immediately. "Brent, I have to be honest with you here." Then I blurted it out: "I do not have financing approved on the house!"

He could sense the anguish in my voice and was empathetic. I told him my complete situation and he calmly said, "Here, give this guy a call. I have seen this broker pull off some tight situations in the past."

I called the guy immediately and explained the situation. He told me up front that this was a stretch and that he would not make any promises. I sent him the paperwork immediately, along with letters detailing why I had so much debt and what I was doing about it.

Very shortly, he found a lender who took some compassion on my situation. The fact that I was being responsible and paying off debt encouraged them. The only problem was that they were going to require 20 percent down and a high interest rate. At this point, we didn't have a penny to our name. Once again Katy and I agreed that we would not ask for help from anyone. I was honest with the broker and he with the lender. The fact that I had paid off two of our credit cards after the sale of our California condo should have helped our credit score, but nothing showed yet. The broker suggested that if we could somehow pay off one more credit card, he could do a quick update on my credit score, and if we reached a certain score, he could possibly get us a 5 percent down loan. That sounded a lot better even though it was still a major stretch.

Meanwhile, back in California, bringing home a new baby and dealing with strife in Katy's family, we had to move out of the condo so the new owners could take possession. So there we were headed in our van back to Portland with no place to call home. We decided it was best for Katy to stay with her parents, even with the discord, while I pursued the house deal and started work at company headquarters. Fortunately, my old boss and his wife let me stay with them at their home. This way I was able to save money toward paying off an additional credit card.

It wasn't easy returning to my workplace in Oregon after being away for three years. There were plenty of power struggles, and I basically had to start at the bottom again. I had to trust the Lord to work all things out for my good. The new management was under a lot of pressure to perform and meet budgets, so I became a target for hour reduction or a possible pay cut. I knew I could not afford a pay cut, so I kept on performing my duties efficiently and effectively to make sure no one could criticize my work. I didn't try to hide my faith either, which made me more of a target than others. I simply stayed focused on the Lord and on my job and stayed away from power struggles.

Learning to Lean on God, Not My Emotions

Then the announcement came about a new manager taking over and several key people being terminated. The rest of us would be re-evaluated to see if we still fit well. My interview was scheduled on a Tuesday at 3:00. I showed up a bit early—this new guy already had a reputation of being a tough player. In a conference call to the entire staff he said, "It's time to separate the wheat from the chaff." I'm sure he didn't know this was a biblical concept to test what is real. R. J. was an intelligent, self-made man who loved to intimidate and be in control. Of course, I came to realize that this was all a front, but nonetheless, at the time, I was a little intimidated. His tongue did not hesitate to say what was on his mind. So there I was sitting at my desk at 2:30, waiting for my interview. Four o'clock rolled around. Five o'clock. Six o'clock. Finally I caught him in the hallway. "Oh good," I said, "I was looking for you. Are we planning on meeting soon?"

He replied, "I wasn't looking for you, but if you want to hang out a while longer I should be finished soon."

"No problem," I said. "Not in any rush."

I sat there and prayed for wisdom, guidance, direction, and protection. Seven o'clock. Eight o'clock. He finally popped his head out the door at 8:30. "I have a couple of minutes for you."

I began to tell him about my background, but he cut me off,

saying he already knew my background. Then I felt the Holy Spirit strengthen me. "R. J.," I said, "I'm here because I believe in our product and believe that it makes a difference in people's lives. I'm a hard worker, I know my stuff, and I only want to be here if I make a difference to the company, including the bottom line. I work on a month-to-month contract. Thus, if ever I'm not happy or if I do not perform for the company, it's 'Adios amigo!'"

R. J. sat back in his chair and said, "Okay, we're on the same wavelength—I'll see you at work tomorrow."

I left feeling empowered and certain that God wanted me to still be with the company. Over the next weeks and months, all of my colleagues in the technical department were let go. The Lord had directed me to secure a place in sales.

Meanwhile, I contacted the mortgage broker who said that he needed the funds immediately to close that one extra credit card. I had saved up a little but was still significantly short to pay it off. All Saturday I fasted and prayed, looking for God's direction. Sunday morning on my way to church my dad called. "Hey kid, how's that house deal going along?" I told him the credit card situation and he said, "I have someone who wants to talk to you." It was his wife, Fengy.

"How much are you short?" she asked.

I told her and then proceeded to say, "But Katy and I...."

She cut me off. "Don't ask or say anything," she said. "I'm wiring the funds tomorrow. You can pay me back in the future. You need a home for your family, and a new baby boy is good luck."

Fengy is an extremely interesting, intelligent, successful business woman whose background in China led her to have Buddhist beliefs. She also studied numerology and learned from her mother, who was a spy in China, to read facial features as a way of assessing a person's character and financial potential. She had also been a Mormon for many years of her life. I do not agree with her beliefs and yet I find her to be open and honest and genuine in her pursuit to understand life spiritually. I am grateful for her friendship and to the fact that God used her in this situation.

Grace, Grace, and More Grace—God Is Good

The sermon that morning was about God's grace and mercy—His pouring out of His blessings on us even though we do not deserve them. How timely! I was in tears through the whole sermon. When I excitedly called Katy to tell her the good news that we had the money, to my surprise she became angry with me. "I thought we agreed that we would not ask for help from anyone!"

"But honey," I said, "you don't understand! I didn't ask for anything! In fact, I was told not to speak."

Finally she calmed down and said, "So I can come back to Portland soon?"

Hearing the tears in her voice of desperation, I said, "Yes, honey. Come on back as soon as possible. I'll rent a hotel room until we move in."

Move in? What if the credit scores did not improve enough? I still did not have enough for 5 percent down. What if it doesn't work out? I drove by the house, all ready to be lived in and yet it seemed so far away. I prayed over and over again for the Lord's hand of direction and protection but felt a little lost and overwhelmed.

Katy and the kids finally arrived and we unloaded our necessities into the hotel room. I called the loan broker who said he'd run the credit score by the end of the following week. "Can't we do it sooner?" I asked. No, we needed time for the new scores to process.

The hotel room was not cheap, and we were trying to save every penny toward the down payment of our house. One of our good friends called and asked if we would like to stay with her for a few days until we moved into our house. We reluctantly, but gladly, accepted.

The next week we anxiously went to meet our broker, joined by my dad and Fengy who were on their way through Portland on a business trip. Desperate, Katy demanded that we get the loan. The mortgage broker looked at her and said, "You know, I don't even know if I can make this happen!"

That was it. Katy broke down, sobbing uncontrollably. My dad tried to take charge with the mortgage broker, but he looked at Dad and said, "I don't know if you know how bad your son's credit is. If you and your wife have the credit and income, you might want to sign for the loan!" This was out of the question for Katy and me, and I said, "Let's get the credit score today, and if I'm approved, great. If not, we will move on." Surrendering everything to God is very freeing!

By this time, Friday afternoon, it was too late to run a credit score, and the broker was leaving on vacation until Tuesday. I felt foolish, helpless, and lost. "Maybe you can't afford this," Dad counseled. "Have you really thought about it?" When I told him that I believe God led me to get this place and I'll continue to put my trust in Him, Dad and Fengy looked at each other like I had lost my mind but had little else to say. "Before you leave," I said, "let's go see the house."

As soon as we got there and were walking toward the front door, Fengy began uttering, "I can't believe it, I can't believe it."

"What!" I said.

"The address is the best number! In Chinese numerology it means forever prosperous!" She then said, "Okay, I believe you; God must be blessing you if you get this house!"

When they departed, I was left with my distraught, angry, and disillusioned wife who still wanted to run away from everyone and everything. It was a miserable night. But during the night God gave me a vision of us all standing at the door of our new house with key in hand. I continued praying and was deeply thankful for the vision. All of a sudden my doubts and anxiety lifted. I had complete peace and shared with Katy what I saw. A little skeptical but slightly encouraged, she was able to pull herself together until Tuesday.

The broker pulled the score Tuesday and by Wednesday he called with congratulations! And he had more good news. "The lender is willing to give you a zero down mortgage if you pay off one more bill!" We gathered every last penny and had just enough to pay off the bill. Two days before my daughter's sixth birthday, we stood at our door in prayer and thanksgiving, exactly as in the vision I had the week before!

Not long after this we found a new church called Solid Rock Fellowship that felt right to both of us. God poured out His blessing on us with new friends and dedicated pastors who love us and pray for us on a regular basis. God has blessed me at my work and has given me favor to contribute creatively to the success of our company. He has also blessed me with patients that I am able to help in this truly integrated approach.

Except for the Problems, Things Are Now Great

And, yes, other than our mortgage we're now debt free! (Well, as I'm now editing this book, I have to confess I fell into a few more traps and got into debt again. Nothing like before and nothing that God cannot handle—will I ever learn?)

Although the stress was excruciatingly painful, I can tell you honestly that every bit was necessary to grow and shape us into the people we are becoming. After reading my testimony you may ask, is God really in the business of real estate? The truth is that God wants to be involved in every area of our lives and will use all kinds of circumstances, both good and bad, to get our attention and to grow our faith! I now have a deeper faith and trust in the Lord. I am more sensitive to things of the Spirit and recognize more fully my daily need for God's provisions, protection, blessings, and grace and mercy. Staying tuned in takes faith and obedience and, even more so, God's faithfulness toward me, despite my flaws. Through tears and trials, I've learned that nothing comforts the heart but God.

St away from the love of money; be satisfied with what you have. For God has said, "I will never fail you. I will never forsake you." That is why we can say with confidence, "The Lord is my helper, so I will not be afraid. What can mere mortals do to me?"[20]

---

[20] Hebrews 13:5-6 New Living Translation

CHAPTER 2
Thriving Spiritually

2.1 What Are You Waiting For?

God, grant me the serenity to accept the things I cannot change;
courage to change the things I can; and
the wisdom to know the difference.
Living one day at a time;
enjoying one moment at a time;
accepting hardship as the pathway to peace.
Taking, as He did, this sinful world as it is, not as I would have it.
Trusting that He will make all things right, if I surrender to His will.
That I may be reasonably happy in this life,
and supremely happy with Him forever in the next.[21]

I f you truly understand and apply the Serenity Prayer, you are well on your way to thriving spiritually. Like the prayer, it all begins with God. ***"And the Lord God formed man of the dust of the ground, and breathed into his nostrils the breath of life; and man became a living soul."***[22]

---

[21] The Serenity Prayer, written by Reinhold Niebuhr
[22] Genesis 2:7 King James Version

This "breath of life" God breathed, is what gave us life. We are spiritual beings because God made us that way. You'll find a plethora of self-help "spirituality" books in the market today, each claiming to know the answers to the universal questions regarding the meaning of life, our purpose, our happiness, and what happens to us after death. Any book that does not point to God and His Word alone as the only source for the answers to these questions is misleading.

The Bible teaches us what it means to be spiritual beings having a human experience. In fact, God is a spiritual being who Himself became human in order to accomplish that which we could not—a life without sin. Originally, God created us in His likeness and image with the ability to think, to create, to love, to feel emotions, and to choose. As we will explore in this chapter, that image of God became distorted after the fall of Adam and Eve. The most important aspect of spirituality is our ability to have a healthy relationship with God Himself. God knew the risks in making us spiritual beings. He knew that we would have the ability not only to choose Him but also to reject Him—to make ourselves out to be little gods (with big egos). Fortunately, God is and has always been in control; He had a perfect plan!

Even our spirituality toward God can be egocentric. We can get so caught up in our own wants and desires that we forget God wants us to die to self and commands us to love one another. Thus the Serenity Prayer helps us to qualify thriving spiritually as being reasonably happy in this lifetime. Even if we are doing great personally, we are called to have compassion for those who are in pain or suffering. God calls us to grieve with those who are grieving and rejoice with those who are rejoicing. Thus, thriving spiritually in this present life must be in the context that we understand there is a purpose for pain and suffering—both for ourselves and for others—and that ultimately we must do our small part to help alleviate it for others who are less fortunate than ourselves. No matter how bad or good things are for you currently, there is always someone else who could use your helping hand. This is especially true for those without a voice in this society—namely, the unborn child, the sick and dying, the handicapped, and the poor.

2.2 Back to Eden

Life was good for Adam and Eve—the luscious garden, communication with God, creativity, joy, health, and love. How did it go so wrong? Was it Eve's fault? Was it Adam's? Was it a set-up by God? Was it satan? Was it meant to happen?

Pain, illness, struggling to make a living, aging, jealousy, envy, pride, and then death. What a great deal that was! Some would argue that if we did not know the ugliness in life we would never fully appreciate the beauty. Maybe there is some truth to that, but I'd have to say from my observations that most of us too easily justify the horrible choices and dark thoughts in our lives. We accept the good and the bad that is now a part of all of us. As a result our lives have become gray. We are less able to discern that which is best! God wants the best for His children but we often settle for the good, the bad, and the ugly.

As I have gotten closer to God personally, I have become more aware of my own faults in the bright light of His holiness. Nothing less than God's holiness is our measuring stick, lest we become conceited and believe that we are better than others or simply good people. Thus the Bible says, *"Stop judging others, and you will not be judged. For others will treat you as you treat them. Whatever measure you use in judging others, it will be used to measure how you are judged. And why worry about a speck in your friend's eye when you have a log in your own?"*[23]

So whether we try to blame Adam and Eve or question why God put the tree of the knowledge of good and evil in the center of the garden in the first place (Isn't that blaming God?), the fact remains that we all inherited a corrupted "gene" called sin. No matter how religious, no matter how wholesome in appearance, no matter what attempts we make to purify ourselves, we cannot change this fact. That is why we all need a Savior. That is why God became human flesh, lived a sinless life, and died on the cross, shedding His innocent blood so that we could be forgiven, redeemed, and spiritually restored. That is why we all need to

---

[23] Matthew 7:1-3 New Living Translation

choose to surrender our ego and put God at the center of our lives. No other decision in your life can come remotely close in significance to receiving God in your heart and surrendering your ego to Him. This decision determines your eternal destiny and your present potential for peace, joy, and happiness. No matter how good you perceive your life to be at this time, it is nothing compared to what God has in store for those who love Him.

If good things are all that God has to offer you, or anyone else, then why do so many people have a problem surrendering their lives to Him? Perhaps you see giving up control of your life as a weakness. From the ego's perspective, this is definitely true. From God's perspective, however, life without Him is foolish, empty, and painful. Perhaps you think that the spiritual life is boring. In my experience, it's anything but boring, and if you are honest with yourself, I think you will agree that the momentary "fun" of sinful activities leaves you empty and dry.

Some people blame hypocrisy—within a church, a priest, a pastor, an evangelist, and Christians as a whole—for their refusal to surrender to God. Others' sinful actions and poor behaviors are certainly not a good reflection of God, but God is still God—perfect and true—and we are still human—sinful and deceitful. Comparing yourself to others can make you look pretty good. Sure, you've made a few mistakes—you're human after all—but when the scales are tipped, your goodness and good deeds certainly outweigh the bad. If there is a heaven, surely you deserve to get there, don't you? I don't mean to challenge your sainthood, but no, you don't. If your family and friends gathered around the television to watch a video revealing all of your thoughts, motivations, and behavior when no one was looking, they would see "Guilty!" written on your forehead. Sin permeates our nature, and none of us can come even remotely close to the perfection required by God in order to enter heaven.

Examine Jesus

Perhaps you believe in God, but have major issues when it

comes to Jesus Christ. Yes, you have heard that Jesus is God, that He left heaven and became human, and that He is part of the mysterious Holy Trinity—one God in three persons, Father, Son, and Holy Spirit. But you have a hard time believing this is true.

Maybe you're willing to believe that Jesus was a prophet, but the Son of God or God Himself, you just can't accept. The Bible claims that Jesus lived a perfect life, that He died on the cross as the perfect sacrifice for our sins, and that on the third day He arose from the grave. But you weren't there—how can anyone know this is true? Well, if Jesus was indeed a prophet, would He have lied to His followers? Josh McDowell, a former skeptic who has examined the life of Jesus, wrote in one of his books, "A prophet cannot be a liar and still be considered a prophet." Jesus said, *"I am the way and the truth and the life. No one comes to the Father except through me."*[24] Even for a prophet, this was an outrageous claim, even blasphemy, to the religious leaders of that time who wanted to kill Him as a violator of their law—unless it is true.

Is it true?

If you have not done so already, I challenge you to examine the life of Jesus for yourself. Many scholars and skeptics who have done this honestly have come to the conclusion that Jesus was and is who He said He is.

2.3 Religion Versus Relationship

Maybe it's organized religion that turns you off to God. You would rather consider yourself an enlightened "spiritual" person open to the many different spiritual perspectives. I took this path for a short time and quickly found myself empty and unsatisfied in my soul. I soon figured out that the Bible is not a religious book at all, nor is God a religion. Since I have experienced a relationship with God, His Word has become like a love letter to me, my owner's manual for living a better life. The Bible is filled with

---

[24] John 14:6

jewels and facts that help me understand God better. In this day and age of spiritualism, we are bombarded by half truths and partial truths that make it difficult to discern what is real. When we come to realize that Truth is a person, Jesus Christ, we can begin to move beyond vain philosophies and self-centered interpretations and really get to the root of understanding the biblical love story.

The Bible is clear that there is no separation between the Word, Jesus, and God. *"In the beginning was the Word, and the Word was with God, and the Word was God. And the Word was made flesh, and dwelt among us (and we beheld his glory, the glory as of the only begotten of the Father), full of grace and truth."*[25] To understand the biblical love story of God reconciling with man, we must look at the gospel in its entirety as God progressively reveals more of his heart and mind to a fallen humanity. The Bible is full of examples of man's desire to be god, man's denial of God and His laws, and man's attempt to create tangible forms of a deity they can see and touch. From the beginning, however, it is only faith that pleases God. Abraham believed in the promises God made to him and the Lord declared him righteous because of his faith.[26]

The Old Testament and the law revealed man's sinful nature and the serious consequences of sin. Animal sacrifice was instituted as a means to teach us that blood (death) is the penalty for sin and requirement for forgiveness. Why? Because that is what God required! God's righteousness demands justice, and sin always has a high price. In the New Testament we come to understand that animal sacrifice was only a foreshadow of the perfect sacrifice, Jesus Christ, the Lamb of God, whose innocent blood is able to cover all our transgressions—past, present, and future. This is part of progressive revelation that God is both loving and just. What appeared to be brutal in the Old Testament— actions such as stoning individuals to death, killing every man, woman, and child in times of war, and sending plagues and death on the Egyptians—underscores the serious consequences of sin.

---

[25] John 1:1, 14 King James Version
[26] See Genesis 15:6

The Bible says, *"For the wages of sin is death, but the gift of God is eternal life in Christ Jesus our Lord."*[27]

This truth—that salvation is a gift from God—separates Christianity from every other religion. Human effort cannot earn favor with God, a ticket to heaven, or eternal life. *"God saved you by his special favor when you believed. And you can't take credit for this; it is a gift from God. Salvation is not a reward for the good things we have done, so none of us can boast about it."*[28]

It does require faith to know God, but not a blind faith. No one can prove to you that anything did or did not happen 2,000 years ago, so if you are inclined to argue the historical content of the Bible, you will find yourself going in circles. What I can tell you rationally, logically, and truthfully is that the person I am becoming through my personal relationship with Jesus Christ is much to my liking. Honesty, courage, humility, patience, and wisdom are just a few of the characteristics that God is building in me. Honestly examining your behaviors, thoughts, and actions can truly help you to see your need for Christ.

Even after examining Jesus with a sincere heart, some people have unanswered questions that are preventing them from making that leap of faith and receiving Christ into their hearts. Often, the longest journey of faith is the distance from the head to the heart. For example, here are some common questions: What about someone who has never heard the name of Jesus Christ? If Jesus really is the only way to God, is this person condemned to hell? If you're concerned about these questions, you obviously have a compassionate heart. Maybe you'll be an evangelist or a missionary someday! The Bible doesn't directly answer these questions, but we know that God is the perfect Judge who will render justice fairly and correctly according to each person's knowledge.

Other common questions are: What about the sincere Buddhist, Hindu, Muslim, or other religious person who's following a different path to God? Can God really deny them entrance into

---

[27] Romans 6:23
[28] Ephesians 2:8-9 New Living Translation

heaven? Well, if they're trying to work their way to heaven, we've already read that the Bible says that's impossible. Once again, we have to say that only God knows their hearts, and we cannot begin to fathom the depth of His love, grace, and mercy. None of us who believe deserve God's grace and salvation in the first place. For you personally, however, is it worth taking the risk of eternal separation from God when you have the free will to choose to believe in God and have eternal life? I hope not! I would never want to scare you into making the most important decision of your life, but better that fear drives you to receive Jesus Christ than to never get around to trusting Him at all!

Knocking at the Door

Regardless, if you are not ready yet to take the step of faith to accept Jesus Christ as your personal Savior, then be honest. I would, however, encourage you to pray this prayer if you are struggling with disbelief:

"God, I honestly do not even know if You exist. My heart, however, is open and desires to know the truth. If You are real, please let me know without doubt in my heart that this is so. I want to be honest with myself and I do not want to follow anyone blindly."

If you prayed this prayer and truly meant it, God will honor your search to know Him. *"You will seek me and find me,"* God says, *"when you seek me with all your heart."*[29] The Lord rewards those who earnestly seek Him.[30] *"Keep on asking, and you will be given what you ask for. Keep on looking, and you will find. Keep on knocking, and the door will be opened. For everyone who asks, receives. Everyone who seeks, finds. And the door is opened to everyone who knocks."*[31] By praying this prayer you are knocking at the door, and God promises in His Word that He will

---

[29] Jeremiah 29:13
[30] See Hebrews 11:6
[31] Matthew 7:7-8

open it! More likely you will find God knocking at the door of your heart if you are seeking the truth. Then, if you invite Him in, He will come in and begin a relationship with you.

My experience in Ontario (when I received baptism by the Holy Spirit) was so real that I had to make my decision right away. I could either lie to myself that it never happened, try to block it out of my mind (denial), or accept that God was real and that He desired to have a personal relationship with me. Obviously, I chose the latter, and I can honestly tell you it was the best decision I have ever made.

God's grace, mercy, and love continue to amaze me, and it is truly my privilege to share the Good News with anyone who is willing to listen. As I write this, tears trickle down my face as I reflect on the many times God has reached out to me—through His Word, through His undeserved blessings, through a friend He sent to my aid when I was in the valley of discouragement, doubt, and denial. I am even thankful for the storms that have purified and strengthened me. I am especially appreciative of the prayers that other believers have offered up on my behalf and for my family, and for the gift of the Holy Spirit, my Helper, who is making me a better husband to my wife, father to my children, and friend to my friends. Most importantly, I am thankful that God is molding and shaping me into the image of His Son so that He can use me for even greater works that He prepared for me before I was even born!

Has God been knocking on the door of your heart? He won't force His way in. Now is the time to exercise faith and invite Him in. You'll never truly be tuned in to God until God is at home in your heart.

As you will come to know, God transcends cultural, financial, personal, and religious differences and knocks on the door of hearts that are seeking to know truth, purpose, and meaning in life. Occasionally, He even goes to extremes to get the attention of people who are running from Him or resisting His plan. Consider Saul of Tarsus, a Christian-hater who met God on the road to Damascus in a blinding light from heaven and the voice of the Lord, received Jesus, and was renamed Paul (see Acts 9:1-31).

There have probably been numerous believers who have prayed for you to make the most important decision of your life—to receive Jesus as your Savior. Here are a couple of true-life testimonies that I hope will encourage you:

Shahab's Story

I met Shahab while playing racquetball and was pleasantly surprised when he identified himself as a Christian. He told me, "I had to hit rock bottom before I was ready to cry out to the Lord." Shahab agreed to let me share his story.

Shahab was born and raised in Pakistan. His dad was a commercial airline pilot and his mother a homemaker. He was the youngest of five siblings, who were all sent to a boarding school at a young age. There, Shahab excelled in sports and academics. Islam was a part of his education, and he soon learned to do the Islamic prayers five times daily. Growing up in a religious family, Shahab says he always had a natural curiosity and healthy desire to learn about God.

When he was 13 years old, Shahab went to visit his brother, who was studying computer science in Arkansas. Shahab enjoyed his time in America, so he asked his parents for permission to stay and pursue his education as well. They agreed, and Shahab began his studies at a Baptist college where he quickly resumed his former routines in sports and academics. For no particular reason, however, he discontinued his prayer life.

Not long after starting school, a new friend, Brandon, began to ask him about his religion. Shahab openly shared with him his Islamic beliefs. Brandon told Shahab with sincerity, "I don't want you to go to hell. I like you." Shahab immediately put up a wall (as I'm sure most people would, when the gospel is shared in such a confrontational way) and told his friend he was just fine—and had a few good laughs about it. Other people would try to approach him, but he had his standard answers and really didn't care about their concern for his soul.

Shahab's world was fine...until he met Sara. Sara grabbed

ahold of his heart and he was like mush before her—his first real love. Shahab made plans to follow his brother to Oregon to continue his education. Just before he moved west, however, Sara dropped a bombshell: She was pregnant. Shahab tried his best to be supportive and commit to being a father and husband, but their relationship fell apart and Sara became more and more distant. Eventually came the shocker: Sara married another man.

That was the end of the rope emotionally for Shahab. He spiraled down into a life of sex and drugs, willing to do anything to numb his pain. Five years whirled by and yet it felt as if the pain of the whole event happened yesterday. One day, Shahab decided to do a little detective work to see if he could track down Sara. He found out she was divorced and living with her parents. He felt in his heart that God was giving him another opportunity. Anxious and hopeful, with his heart pounding, Shahab called Sara at home. Her dad answered the phone. Without a pause, Shahab said, "Is Sara there please?"

For what felt like an eternity, there was silence. Then he heard her familiar voice. "Sara, how are you?"

She did not recognize the voice. "Don't you remember?" he said. "This is Shahab."

Sara was surprised, but seemed glad to hear his voice. Before long, she sent him pictures of his daughter and was willing to meet in Oregon. Much like a romance novel, Shahab married his first love. Unfortunately, the honeymoon phase came to a sudden stop when a woman called their house claiming that Shahab was the father of her child. Although Shahab believed the woman was lying, Sara moved back in with her parents, but only after scaring Shahab by swallowing an overdose of Paxil.

Shahab was not ready to give up, however, and even though he began using drugs again, he ended up moving in with Sara and her parents. Things actually started to improve, but on a trip to Oregon with Sara, Shahab discovered some e-mails that indicated Sara was flirting with another man. Devastated, Shahab considered suicide and began to plan the dramatic conclusion: He would fly back to Sara's home with a pistol. When she opened the door he would say "Happy birthday" and then shoot himself.

Meanwhile, Shahab's sister in Nevada was having marital troubles of her own. Shahab decided he would do one last gesture of goodwill for his sister before ending his life. It was Easter Sunday. Shahab had no money but was determined to go to Las Vegas to help his sister move out of her situation. Sara worked for the airlines, and Shahab begged her to get him on a flight to Vegas. The odds were overwhelmingly impossible, but miraculously he made it on the last flight out.

One of Shahab's friends had given him a Bible, and on this fateful flight to Las Vegas Shahab opened the book and began to connect with it for the first time. He cried out in his heart, "Jesus, if You are real, help me. Be my Savior. Save me!" As he read about Jesus' crucifixion, he began to weep uncontrollably. He kept asking, "Why did they do this to You, Jesus? Why?" On that plane, thousands of feet in the air, Shahab had an encounter with his Savior.

Almost two years later, when Shahab recalls the messed-up man he used to be, he understands his need for God's love, grace, and mercy! He prays for another chance with Sara and his daughter, this time based on the Rock, Jesus Christ.

Julie's Story (in Her Own Words)

Growing up, nobody ever dreams of having a life marked by loss and grief. I certainly didn't. I lived a simple childhood. Mom was a dedicated housewife, always home and available for my sisters and me. Dad worked in corporate America to provide for his family. My parents taught us kids from the Bible daily. In fact, God was such a part of my upbringing that I would play "church" just as much as "house." With my stuffed animals lined up in front of me, I'd teach them worship songs and Bible lessons. God was the center of my family's home.

In middle school, however, I began to question everything I had been taught, what I believed, and if I really was a Christian. Although there were times of intense confusion, I didn't tell anybody about my uncertainty.

My life changed drastically when I was 14. Mom, my source of security and love, was diagnosed with terminal cancer. Suddenly, fear invaded my simple life. I feared losing my mom. I feared what would happen to my family. But even more, I feared God. All my questions about what I believed became so much more real and deep.

My fears intensified when my friend was killed in a car accident a year later. I remember sitting at her funeral, with my dying mom sitting two chairs down from me, thinking about how short and uncertain this life is. Just days before, I was able to laugh and share emotions with my friend, and now it was all over. I knew in my heart that there was something more, but that scared me, too.

Coming home from church a couple of months later, these thoughts becoming more and more frequent, I found Mom resting on the living room couch and in a lot of pain. There were questions I needed to ask before she died, just so I wouldn't have to wonder when she was gone. "Mom, are you scared to die?" (I asked this because I myself was terrified.)

"No, I am not at all scared to die," she said. Then she looked at me and continued, "But I can only die in peace if I know that you girls will be there with me. Can you tell me that you *know* you will be with me in heaven, Julie?"

I remember feeling this overwhelming sense of adrenaline run through my body. I didn't know.

That question turned into a couple of hours of conversation with my mom and dad. Dad took me to 1 John 5:11-13, which states, ***"And this is the testimony: God has given us eternal life, and this life is in his Son. He who has the Son has life; he who does not have the Son of God does not have life. I write these things to you who believe in the name of the Son of God so that you may know that you have eternal life."*** It was then that I realized I could know, with full assurance, that I could spend eternity in heaven. It was all in Jesus. Up to that point, I had been told about Jesus Christ and did all the things I had been told I should do, but I didn't know Him personally. That day I told the Lord that I needed Him to save me. I didn't just want to claim the name of Jesus nominally anymore. I wanted, I needed, to *know*

Him personally. I told God that I had been living off my parents' faith; now it was my own.

A couple of years later Mom would go to be with Jesus. It still amazes me that she is with Him now. She actually sees His face. And even though she is not with me, I have hope. I know, with certain expectation, that I will see my mom again. And as she introduced the person of Jesus to me here on earth, she just might introduce Him to me again when I am one day with her, but this time face to face.

It is true that I have had much brokenness I never anticipated as a child. Since mom died nine years ago, my uncle and grandpa have also died. Right now a woman who has been a mother figure to me in recent years is dying of the same cancer that took my mom's life. But I can thank the Lord. I'm learning that this life is not all about my happiness. It is about Jesus Christ—about knowing Him, loving Him, and being made like Him. He knew that this is what I needed in order to surrender my life to Him. So as much as I loved my mom and as much as she loved me, neither of us would do it differently. I think of a passage I memorized when I was in the waiting room at one of Mom's radiation appointments years ago: *"Therefore we do not lose heart. Though outwardly we are wasting away, yet inwardly we are being renewed day by day. For our light and momentary troubles are achieving for us an eternal glory that far outweighs them all. So we fix our eyes not on what is seen, but on what is unseen. For what is seen is temporary, but what is unseen is eternal."*[32]

Throughout the years, I have often tried to go by a formula as to how to be spiritually mature. But in the end it is all about faith in Christ. It is not faith in a concept or theory but in the *person* of Jesus. We need to choose faith today and do it again tomorrow and the next day. Then even when it is just a decision, and the emotions only follow, we can look back and see how we have grown closer to Jesus. And we know Him as good. We don't need to try to convince Him to be good. He just is. That is His nature.

---

[32] 2 Corinthians 4:16-18

2.4 The Origins of Ego

I hope at this point you have already surrendered your ego and given your life to Jesus like Shahab and Julie and I have. If not, perhaps understanding the origins of the ego will help put things further into perspective.

Ego has a long history, going all the way back to the beginning of creation. Lucifer, one of the most beautiful angels in heaven, was the first to rebel against God and thus is the father of ego. The prophet Isaiah in the Bible's Old Testament gives us a glimpse of Lucifer's heart:

You said in your heart,
"I will ascend to heaven;
I will raise my throne above the stars of God;
I will sit enthroned on the mount of assembly,
on the utmost heights of the sacred mountain.
I will ascend above the tops of the clouds;
I will make myself like the Most High."[33]

It was satan (the fallen angel, Lucifer) who, back in the Garden of Eden, deceived our first human mother, Eve, and our first human father, Adam, into rebellion against God. God had created a perfect environment for His wonderful creation to live in, and the man and woman enjoyed an intimate relationship with Him. They weren't robots, however. God created Adam and Eve with a free will, with the capacity to choose to love God and obey Him or to reject God and disobey Him. God created Adam and Eve in His image to enjoy a relationship with them, but He would not force them to love Him.

Of course, God knew that evil already existed, but as long as His new creations chose to obey Him, He could protect them from it. In the Garden of Eden God made every type of tree and fruit that were pleasing to the eye and mouth. And the Lord God commanded the man, saying, *"Of every tree of the garden you*

---

[33] Isaiah 14:13-14

*may freely eat; but of the tree of the knowledge of good and evil
you shall not eat, for in the day that you eat of it you shall surely
die."*[34] This was the only requirement man had to follow in order
to enjoy all of God's blessings.

Satan had a different agenda—to deceive the man and woman
God loved:

*Now the serpent was more cunning than any beast of the field
which the LORD God had made. And he said to the woman, "Has
God indeed said, 'You shall not eat of every tree of the garden'?"
And the woman said to the serpent, "We may eat the fruit of the
trees of the garden; but of the fruit of the tree which is in the
midst of the garden, God has said, 'You shall not eat it, nor shall
you touch it, lest you die.'" Then the serpent said to the woman,
"You will not surely die. For God knows that in the day you eat
of it your eyes will be opened, and you will be like God, knowing
good and evil."*[35]

We all know the outcome of Eve's choice. The desire and
obsession for self-love, self-realization, and self-glorification—in
other words, ego—has continued ever since. Satan still uses the
same tactics to destroy lives today:

1. Creating doubt about God's Word.
2. Denying or reducing the consequences of sin.
3. Tempting our minds and human nature with sin's pleasures.
4. Encouraging us to think we are the masters of our own
   destiny—boosting our egos!

A few things should not be overlooked in this exchange
between the serpent and Eve. First of all, the serpent was actually
talking! Can animals talk? Eve's reaction, or rather lack of
reaction, to the serpent talking would seem to indicate that indeed
animals did talk before the first humans sinned, an event known as

---

[34] Genesis 2:16-17 New King James Version
[35] Genesis 3:1-5 New King James Version

the Fall. Why do I even bring this up? Because if you read this initially without understanding this possibility, you may have thought this sounded like a fairy tale. It is not! Events in the Bible occurred in the past as written. The creation of Adam and Eve and their fall into sin are not fables or fiction, but part of the true history of the world and a love story that is still unfolding. God doesn't answer all of our questions about history, but in the most important areas He is very clear and serious.

Second, the serpent was not a snake as we see in the typical cartoon depictions of man's original sin. The Bible refers to the serpent as one of the more subtle beasts that the Lord God had created. The serpent may have been satan taking the form of this beast himself, but more likely it was satan manipulating or using the serpent to accomplish his deceit.

Did Adam and Eve actually die after eating of this fruit? No, they didn't die physically as if the fruit were poisoned. They died spiritually. They became ashamed of their bodies, experienced pain and conflict, and felt alienated from God. Eventually they would die physically and, apart from God implementing His magnificent plan of salvation, risk eternal separation from God. It is interesting to note that no person in biblical history actually lived to be a thousand years old, which is referred to as one day in heaven.

"But, beloved, do not forget this one thing, that with the Lord one day is as a thousand years, and a thousand years as one day."[36]

Regardless, we are all going to die because of Adam and Eve's disobedience. Sin is in our genetic makeup (spiritual DNA) and we cannot overcome it through our own power. The prophet Jeremiah stated it clearly when he said:

Can the Ethiopian change his skin
or the leopard its spots?
Neither can you do good
who are accustomed to doing evil.[37]

---

[36] 2 Peter 3:8 New King James Version
[37] Jeremiah 13:23

Discipline will not work, will power does not last, and self-help books cannot change your heart. Jesus said, ***"Without me you can do nothing."***[38]

Obviously there are varying degrees of sin with varying degrees of consequences. Sins such as pride, love of money, envy, and lust are common to our society. The problem with sin, no matter how small our error may be, is that it tends to have a snowball effect. For example, what may start off as an "innocent" lie can turn into a habitual pattern and eventually lead to bigger lies even to people we care about the most. The sins of ego and pride never allow us to humble ourselves enough to recognize our error and to truly seek help.

How can we overcome sin? When we receive Jesus Christ as our Savior, our sins are completely forgiven—past, present, and future. Unfortunately, we still have our sin nature even after we are saved, and thus will battle with it until we are given our new spiritual, incorruptible bodies in heaven. The good news is that if we confess our sins God will be faithful and just to forgive us of all of our sins and purify us from all unrighteousness (see 1 John 1:9).

When we receive Christ, He gives us the power of His Holy Spirit to overcome our daily temptations, to transform us into His own image, and to give us victory over our adversary, the devil. Satan's goal is to steal, manipulate, and destroy that which God has promised to all of His children. In doing so he hopes to distort God's image in order to deceive as many people as he can. Satan is the master of deception and the father of lies.

The Perfect Sacrifice

Why was it necessary for Jesus to die in our place? In the Old Testament it was common practice to sacrifice a perfect animal as an offering for the sins of the people. The blood of the innocent animal would pay the penalty for various sins. God accepted those sacrifices even though they were temporary and imperfect. In other

---

[38] John 15:5 New King James Version

words, there has always been a cost for sin that someone had to pay. In the Bible, animal sacrifices were actually the foreshadowing of the ultimate and perfect sacrifice, which needed to be done only once. That sacrifice was Jesus, *"The Lamb of God, who takes away the sin of the world!"*[39] He came in human form—conceived by the overshadowing of the Holy Spirit upon the virgin Mary—overcame all temptations, lived a sin-free life, and most important of all, He conquered death. The price that Jesus paid for us on the cross can never be measured. It is purely God's grace and love that allows us to be declared "not guilty" and as clean as a pure white snow. If we can comprehend that glorious thought that all of our sins were nailed to the cross—that Jesus paid it all—we will never be the same again. For more than a century, Christians have sung the words of a much loved hymn, "It Is Well With My Soul":

My sin, oh, the bliss of this glorious thought!
My sin, not in part but the whole,
Is nailed to the cross, and I bear it no more,
Praise the Lord, praise the Lord, O my soul!

The apostle Paul wrote, *"Therefore if any man be in Christ, he is a new creature: old things are passed away; behold, all things are become new."*[40] "Are become new"—that's in the present tense. In other words, Christ is continually renewing us if we allow Him to. Therefore, even if you have accepted Jesus Christ as your Savior in the past, He continues to free you from your sinful nature in the present. *"But to all who believed him and accepted him, he gave the right to become children of God. They are reborn! This is not a physical birth resulting from human passion or plan—this rebirth comes from God."*[41]

Perhaps you, or someone you know, accepted Jesus Christ several years ago and lived on a spiritual high for days or weeks on end. Over time, however, you became caught up with the cares of

---

[39] John 1:29
[40] 2 Corinthians 5:17 King James Version
[41] John 1:12-13 New Living Translation

the world and perhaps went completely astray. If this is you, do not feel bad. Even the apostle Paul, who was a rock-solid believer, struggled with the tugs and pulls of his sinful human nature. *"For I know that in me (that is, in my flesh) dwelleth no good thing: for to will is present with me; but how to perform that which is good I find not. For the good that I would do, I do not: but the evil which I would not, that I do…. O wretched man that I am! Who shall deliver me from the body of this death? I thank God through Jesus Christ our Lord. So then with the mind I myself serve the law of God; but with the flesh the law of sin."*[42]

Paul continues in this letter in the New Testament to discuss the importance of not giving up and not giving in to sin despite our sinful nature. This is why we must feed ourselves with spiritual food. Having friends that will encourage you in your walk of faith is important as well as regular Bible study, prayer, and worship with other believers.

2.5 Our New Family

Having a personal relationship with Jesus Christ gives us the opportunity to restore our relationship to God as it was before Adam and Eve sinned. Adam and Eve in their disobedience caused death to reign, whereas Mary, in her obedience, received Jesus, through whom we can all be made alive again. The curse of Adam and Eve's sin was broken by what Jesus accomplished on the cross.

This means that when we accept Jesus Christ we can once again have a relationship with our heavenly Father. Unlike our earthly fathers who can and do fail us, our heavenly Father is perfect and faithful to us. When we receive Christ, we are adopted into His heavenly family and become children of the Most High. Jesus even calls us his brothers and sisters and thus, by matter of relationship, we also receive a heavenly mother. What a blessing, what an honor to have the same mother as Jesus! *"Elizabeth gave*

---

[42] Romans 7:18, 19, 24, 25 King James Version

a glad cry and exclaimed to Mary, 'You are blessed by God above all other women, and your child is blessed. What an honor this is, that the mother of my Lord should visit me! When you came in and greeted me, my baby jumped for joy the instant I heard your voice! You are blessed because you believed that the Lord would do what he said.'"[43]

Eve, *"the mother of all the living,"*[44] was disobedient to God. Mary, on the other hand, exercised faith and obedience to God and became our new spiritual mother. *"Near the cross of Jesus stood his mother, his mother's sister, Mary the wife of Clopas, and Mary Magdalene. When Jesus saw his mother there, and the disciple whom he loved standing nearby, he said to his mother, 'Dear woman, here is your son,' and to the disciple, 'Here is your mother.' From that time on, this disciple took her into his home."*[45]

On top of this, everyone who receives Christ becomes our spiritual brother or sister. God wants us to work together to accomplish His work here on earth. In a mystery that we do not fully understand here on earth, even the saints in heaven who have gone before us are part of this family and their prayers continue to ascend to God (see Revelation 8:3-4). Keep in mind that we are only to pray to God. We also can, and are required, to pray with and for one another.

One would think that once we receive Christ everything would be perfect again, just like it was in the Garden of Eden. This is the paradox of the Christian life. Although Christ has already conquered sin and death, we continue to be affected by both until our death or until the final redemption of the world. But as Jesus said, *"I have told you all this so that you may have peace in me. Here on earth you will have many trials and sorrows. But take heart, because I have overcome the world."*[46]

The adversary, satan, continues his effort, along with his host

---

[43] Luke 1:42-45 New Living Translation
[44] Genesis 3:20
[45] John 19:25-27
[46] John 16:33 New Living Translation

of demons, to disrupt our peace. *"Then the dragon became angry at the woman, and he declared war against the rest of her children—all who keep God's commandments and confess that they belong to Jesus."*[47] "The dragon" is satan, and "the woman" is Mary—one of the meanings that Bible scholars give to this passage. The amazing thing about Scripture is that there can be several possible meanings to a particular passage due to the depth of God's Word.

You would think that we would have learned from the grave mistake of Adam and Eve. In fact, it would be convenient to remain in the first stage of our ego and continue to blame Adam and Eve for all of our problems! As we spiritually mature, however, we realize that we must truly allow God into all aspects of our lives on a continual basis and put on "the full armor of God" for protection. *"Put on the full armor of God so that you can take your stand against the devil's schemes. For our struggle is not against flesh and blood, but against the rulers, against the authorities, against the powers of this dark world and against the spiritual forces of evil in the heavenly realms."*[48]

Thus we must not fool ourselves that life is or should be easy, although it is God's desire that we live an "abundant" life filled with meaning and peace (see John 10:10). Only humility, confession, and prayer can keep us safe in the midst of serious spiritual warfare. We need the prayers of our brothers and sisters in Christ to join with the prayers of our foremost Advocate, Jesus Christ. Ultimately, God is Our shield. *"He grants a treasure of good sense to the godly. He is their shield, protecting those who walk with integrity. He guards the paths of justice and protects those who are faithful to Him."*[49] We have our part to play in knowing the Word of God (even Jesus used Scripture when satan came against Him) and in confessing our sins and fleeing from them in true repentance.

---

[47] Revelation 12:17 New Living Translation
[48] Ephesians 6:11-12
[49] Proverbs 2:7-8 New Living Translation

Sin Will Always Have Consequences

The fact remains that there are still consequences for our sin. Sins committed today still disrupt our relationship with God even though all of our past sins have been wiped clean. That is why we often find that certain aspects of our lives are still a mess. I know personally that the one area that I failed to surrender over to God, namely our finances, was the area in which we had the most problems. Although I was willing to surrender all other aspects of my life, I thought I could do a better job than God at managing our finances. Not so! As I have slowly relinquished control and have begun to tithe, God has begun to restore our finances. As a believer with the knowledge I have, I know that I am held more accountable to God's Word. I will never be completely at peace or receive the fullness of God's blessings until I fully trust Him with all aspects of my life. This process involves a daily surrender and requires that we seek God with all our heart, mind, and soul.

Of course, the true test of our faith comes when we are getting closer to the mountaintop. Will we get complacent? Will we start to take things for granted? Will we become prideful? I hope and pray not. We should always seek God and give Him praise in good times and in bad times. We should also seek Him and praise Him for who He is. Remember, even while we were yet sinners living in rebellion and rejection of our Creator, He loved us. God is love. If you and I were the only sinners on this planet, God still would have sent His Son to die for us. In comparison to love this high and wide and deep, His blessings are a mere side benefit.

2.6 The Mountaintop

Symbolically, we can think of the Garden of Eden as being the top of the tallest mountain where our relationship to God is perfect, where the views are spectacular, and where there truly is bliss. This is where Adam and Eve were placed after God created them.

The top of the mountain represents heaven on earth. Adam and Eve had health, abundance, purpose, and most importantly a direct relationship with their Creator.

After their sin, they tumbled all the way down into the valley. The valley represents hell on earth. Since we have all inherited Adam and Eve's sin, we all start our lives living in the valley, the place where we attempt to fill the holes in our hearts that only God can fill. We try to replace God with things such as money, career, relationships, religion, and spirituality, to name a few. Although these things are not necessarily bad in and of themselves, they are simply illusions or mirages if we think we will find lasting peace and happiness in them. It is not until we come to the saving knowledge of what Jesus Christ did for us on the cross at Calvary, believe in Him, and receive Him in our hearts that we come out of the valley to mid-mountain. He takes us out of the valley that represents ego, sin, and death as only He can. Jesus is the only one who conquered original sin by living a completely sin-free life and overcoming death through His resurrection. Once again the beloved hymn captures the reality of this restoration and freedom!

> My sin, oh, the bliss of this glorious thought!
> My sin, not in part but the whole,
> Is nailed to the cross, and I bear it no more,
> Praise the Lord, praise the Lord, O my soul!

Accepting a personal relationship with Jesus Christ puts you in the middle of the mountain. Why not to the top? Because we still live in a fallen world and God wants us to exercise our faith and free will toward him daily so that we can mature, grow, and become more like His Son. The path from the middle of the mountain back down into the valley can happen easily. All we have to do is make a few compromises, surround ourselves with a few negative people, allow our ego to elevate (pride), and allow sin to creep back in. The path to the top of the mountain is straight and narrow. It requires that we bear each cross that God gives us to carry for our purification, for our faith-building, and for our sanctification (becoming holy in God's sight). We also must have victory over each cross by our faith, by our humility, by our obedience to God, and by accepting the gift of the Holy Spirit who gives us the strength we need when we are weak. God never gives us more than we can handle as long as we turn to Him for our strength.

The path back to the top is not easy! Compromised believers are commonplace. God allows us to exercise our free will toward Him or toward our own desires; toward human philosophy or toward biblical realities. We still have to make good decisions, seek understanding from God's perspective, remain humble, and discern between good and evil. *"Trust in the LORD with all your heart, and lean not on your own understanding; in all your ways acknowledge Him, and He shall direct your paths."*[50] Doing this is not our natural inclination even after receiving Christ. Thus, we need to depend on God's grace and mercy to help us live as this proverb advises.

God's Mercy Continues

Even though we are sure to stumble and fall due to our human weaknesses, God's mercy prevails despite the mess we make of our lives. God is in the business of cleaning up the mess! No matter how far we have fallen into the valley, He will pull us out of our misery if we are truly sorry (repentant) for what we have done.

True repentance is when you acknowledge your sin and then turn 180 degrees in the opposite direction. Being sorry has very little meaning when you do not change your direction or keep on repeating the same mistake over and over again. Remember that you must lean on God for strength, wisdom, and understanding in order to overcome your sinful nature, which is sure to take you back into the valley. *"Enter ye in at the strait gate: for wide is the gate, and broad is the way, that leadeth to destruction, and many there be which go in thereat: Because strait is the gate, and narrow is the*

---

[50] Proverbs 3:5-6 New King James Version

way, which leadeth unto life, and few there be that find it."[51]

Obviously, staying on the narrow road is not easy or else everyone would be on it. Doesn't everyone want to receive the fullness of God's blessing during his or her life and into eternity? Health, provisions, peace, romance, joy, a protected family, and eternity with the Creator—who in their right mind would not want all of these things? If you find yourself struggling in one or more areas of your life, it is possible that satan has found an unguarded gateway to infiltrate your life. *"The thief does not come except to steal, and to kill, and to destroy. I have come that they may have life, and that they may have it more abundantly.*"[52] Yes, it is a struggle to keep what God has promised to us. Sin is the perfect open gate that allows our enemy to come in.

And be sure of this: satan is after more than you. He's on the prowl for your family, for your nation, for the entire world, wherever he can destroy or steal what rightfully belongs to God. We in America have been extremely blessed as a nation in so many ways. This country was founded on God's Word. I believe that September 11, 2001, was a heavenly reminder that we need to put God first in America.

This is a letter that the Holy Spirit inspired me to write shortly after the tragedy:

September 19, 2001

To my dear family, friends, and neighbors who are seeking understanding of this recent tragic event, I want to share what God has put in my heart.

Lately we have all heard questions and comments such as, "This was God's will," "Why would a loving God allow such a thing to occur?" or the worse yet, "This was God's judgment on New York."

As a defender of truth and a lover of God, I felt moved to share

---

[51] Matthew 7:13-14 King James Version
[52] John 10:10 New King James Version

this with anyone who is willing to listen and, hopefully, hear God's perspective.

At church last night we were praying, along with millions of other people across the world, for peace to those families who lost loved ones and for everyone else who is grieving throughout this nation and abroad. A preacher spoke a very important message: God is good. If you take an "o" out of good, you don't lose anything, because what you have left is God. However, if you add a "d" to evil, you have the devil. That is who is responsible for this horrific tragedy!

Still you may ask: Why did God allow the devil to influence those involved to commit this awful crime? The answer lies in the fact that God has given us a free will. He allows us to exercise our will for good or for evil, and He allows us to follow Him or the devil. This is the freedom that we fight so hard for in this country that allows people to love God or hate God, to produce good movies or to create pornography, to be pro-life or pro-abortion. God is so merciful that He allows the sun to shine down on both *good* people and *bad* people.

Now there is no doubt that God does bless and protect individuals and nations that love Him and His people. In fact, America has been extremely blessed and protected for many years. Is it possible that His hand of protection has been ever so slightly lifted off of us because of our own evils and sins? We kick God out of our schools, we don't allow Him in public places, we are not horrified at aborting life. We allow pornography to flood our streets and, worst of all, we allow our tax dollars to fund scientists to experiment with God's genetic material from an aborted life. Yes, God's people are at least partly to blame for not speaking out against evil in our own front yard.

A tragedy like this exposes our hearts as a people and as a nation. We are quick to judge, put blame on *innocent* people, are ready and willing to seek revenge, and are even willing to put the blame on God. The reason I highlighted "innocent" and "good" is because God says that we all have sinned and thus no one is innocent. In fact, God says in 2 Peter 3:9 that it is His will that all should repent and none should perish. This includes Jews, Muslims, Christians, Hindus, blacks, whites, yellow, green, rich, and poor—and believe it or not, Osama bin Laden himself.

God loves you and me so much that He was willing to sacrifice His own Son so that our sins could be forgiven. How many of you would be willing to give up your own child for someone else's sins? The sacrificial blood of Jesus (sin-free) covers our own sins completely so that we can regain the relationship that God once had with Adam and Eve before the fall. There is no other name given under heaven by which we can be saved.

So let's all repent and turn to the living God who overcame death itself and who offers us peace, joy, and blessings in this lifetime and through eternity. Love God with all your heart, mind, and soul, and love your neighbor as yourself. Yes, the people that committed this crime need to be brought to justice, but revenge (or vengeance) is God's.

May God bless you all,

Shaun

2.7 The Battle for Your Soul

Am I making too much of the devil? I used to think the devil existed "somewhere out there," but had nothing to do with my life and loved ones.

Then my brother died.

After Steven's tragic death, I embraced my mom and told her how sorry I was. In the house, her husband was on the bed crying uncontrollably. He embraced me and kept repeating "I told him not to drive, I told him not to drive." My little sister, Julia, was in shock and could not say anything. We were all living hell on this earth in those moments.

I sat in silence next to my niece on the porch steps as we observed the tears flowing from friends and family. As I looked up around a vehicle, someone was walking toward us. The hood of his jacket concealed much of his face until he drew closer and looked directly at me. *Am I hallucinating from shock or is that Steven?* Our eyes locked for what seemed minutes but was probably only seconds. I saw my brother's face; he looked terribly sad and yet a peace transcended through my entire body. Still thinking I must be hallucinating, I pinched my cheek and, sure enough, as I looked up it was my brother's best friend. Somewhat relieved, I sat there and reflected on this newfound peace that came over me. Then my niece stated nonchalantly, "I just saw Steven." I looked at her and said, "Oh my God, I just saw him too."

This confirmation was enough that I felt moved to share my "hallucination" with everyone. The mood began to shift in the house. In my mind and soul there was a sense that everything was going to be okay.

That day I had a heart-to-heart talk with my little sister, who revealed some things to me that brought more questions. Two weeks prior to this tragedy, my sister, her friend, and Steven were driving in the evening when they saw a light, a shooting star, flash across the sky. At the end of its trail it left a kind of impression of a bird. Amused, my sister and her friend said, "Cool, did you see that?"

When my sister looked over at my brother, he was crying. She asked him what was wrong. "Something bad is going to happen," he said.

"What are you talking about?" my sister quickly replied.

Steven didn't respond, and Julia dropped the matter. The next day, however, she asked him what he was thinking when they saw that light in the sky. Again he started to cry. My sister didn't know what to say, then told him, "Steven, be careful with your driving and don't do anything stupid."

Just hours after I had this talk with her, I received the funeral brochure. It had a picture of a star, a bird, and some silhouettes of some buildings. Apparently the individuals who did the brochure got the picture over the Internet—it was supposedly the star above Bethlehem. On the second page was a poem entitled "Do Not Grieve for Me." At first glance I didn't think anything of it and put the brochure aside as I helped out with cleaning the house. I had the urge to scrub and clean and enlisted many people to help. By the end of the day we started preparing to paint the outside of the house, a job that had remained unfinished for several years.

Late that evening after I collapsed for a few hours, I sat alone in the living room and picked up the funeral brochure again. Looking at it closely, I wondered, *"What did this all represent? Was there any meaning to this light, to the black bird?"* For the first time I noticed a cross at the bottom of the picture. It seemed a little odd for the cross to be next to the buildings in the ground. Normally a cross would be on top of a church or on top of a hill. As I looked closer at the cross, I noticed it had a pointed end much like a dagger. This definitely set off the alarms in my mind. And the buildings looked like gravestones with this black bird hovering over its targeted prey. Yes, the Holy Spirit revealed to me that this picture represented satan's attempt to claim victory for this tragedy. The poem inside the front cover offered confirmation. "Do not grieve for me," it began. "I am following the path that God laid for me."

That was all I needed to read to realize that this poem was inappropriate for my brother's situation. Does God lay a path of destruction for a teenager 12 hours after a wedding? On top of that, alcohol, speeding, and disobedience to parental authority! Certainly not!

Several teenagers, including my sister, were sitting outside in the dark, still in shock from the course of events. I went outside and showed my sister the picture that had a whole new meaning to me now. I asked her to take a look at it again and to tell me what she thought it represented. She sat for a few minutes and finally blurted out, "I don't know. It just looks rather dark."

"Exactly!" I said. When I pointed out to her all the things in the picture, she immediately said, "Oh my God, I do not like this picture. I don't want it going out to anyone, and I'm going to redesign a new one tonight." This was at 2:00 a.m., just hours before the first funeral service for school friends.

When I read the words of the poem to the teenagers sitting outside, I asked them if they wanted to get to know a God that has a plan similar to what just happened to my brother. Not surprisingly, they all replied no. I told them that likewise I would not want to know a God that had such a plan. There's only one who has a plan to kill, steal, and destroy, and his name is satan. In the next couple of hours we remade the entire brochure with a picture from my brother's graduation and the following words at the bottom:

May God bring Truth and Light to all.
Please learn from my mistakes.
Do not drink and drive,
Do not speed and drive,
Honor and listen to your parents.

These simple words had a profound impact on everyone who read them. There were some who were against this brochure being handed out, but the Holy Spirit used Steven's father, Bill, to stand firmly behind it.

At the church funeral the following day, I asked if I could come up and say a few words. The priest agreed, so I spoke what the Holy Spirit moved me to say:

"As a parent of a precious child that God has entrusted me with, I believe it is important that we defend our children against the evils of the world. Evil comes in many different forms and requires that we monitor the music that our children are listening to, the television and movies that they watch, and even the type of friends that they hang out with.

"I want to explain what I believe happened to my brother. A few weeks prior to this tragedy my brother, sister, and friend were driving in the car when they saw a light flash in the sky and it left the impression of a bird. For whatever reason the thought entered into my brother's mind that something bad was going to happen to him. Instead of questioning that thought or asking for help from his parents or his priest, he tried to deal with it on his own. Instead of it going away, it kept on building up in his thoughts to the point where he was almost obsessed with the thought that something bad was going to happen. In the end he subconsciously (with satan's help) fulfilled that thought by the choices he made. Drinking and driving, speeding, and not wearing a seat belt were not things he would normally do.

"As we all know, thoughts and beliefs can be very powerful both toward the negative and the positive. We must talk with our children more to find out their thoughts. We must spend more quality time with them, and we must pray for the Lord's guidance for our children and for us as parents."

My brother was a well-adjusted and good child. He made a few bad decisions and most importantly he lacked spiritual discernment—the ability to discern that which comes from God versus that which comes from satan.

Developing Discernment

The best way to develop spiritual discernment is to know the truth well. It then becomes simple to discern when something is a fake. When most of us look at a diamond and a zirconium, we are not going to be able to tell the difference. It is only when we look carefully that we are able to see a fake clearly. If satan were so obvious, he would not be able to deceive anyone. Keep in mind that satan was once Lucifer, the most beautiful angel in all of heaven. If he did not appear attractive to anyone, no one would be deceived. Sex, money, power, and lies—satan's tools—have deceived many who may have had the best of intentions but fell to the weakness of their flesh. The best way to overcome the devil is to stay focused on Jesus, on the cross, and to stay in the Word. This is our armor of protection, our strength and our fortress in every situation.

The spiritual battles will continue all of our lives. That is why we must never become weary of doing good or become complacent in our walk. We must move from faith to faith to victory after victory. We need prayer, fellowship with one another, encouragement, study, and correction at times. This is how we grow and mature into the spiritual warriors that God desires us to be. This is a long distance run that we are all in together on the same team. It is a serious game, and yet we can learn to laugh at the enemy in his futile attempts to mess with God's will for His children. In fact, God will take that which was meant for evil and turn it to good for His children.

At times you can chuckle as you clearly watch the enemy try to distract your attempt to share the truth with someone who is open to hear it. The phone will ring, someone will knock at the door, a pager will go off, or numerous other distractions will occur. At other times you may have to just hold on tight and focus on Jesus as the enemy shoots his arrows at you. Regardless of the situation, continue to plant the seeds that may take hold and bear fruit at any given time. Prayer is the water we can continue to pour out to nurture the seeds we have planted. We must always remember, however, that these battles occur in the spiritual realm and that our victories are not our own. Thanks be to God through His Son, Jesus Christ!

So until Jesus returns to earth to set up His kingdom we must persevere and fight the good fight for our present peace and happiness, and for our future glorious life with God. In the next life (for those who are in Christ) there will be no more pain and suffering. There will be reunions with loved ones who have gone before us, and best of all we will see our Creator face to face! These future glories we cannot begin to comprehend!

Until that time, the best prayer we can pray is the one that Jesus taught us, known as the Lord's Prayer:

Our Father which art in heaven, hallowed be thy name. Thy kingdom come, thy will be done in earth, as it is in heaven. Give us this day our daily bread. And forgive us our debts, as we forgive our debtors. And lead us not into temptation, but deliver us from evil: For thine is the kingdom, and the power, and the glory, for ever. Amen.[53]

---

[53] Matthew 6:9-13 King James Version

2.8 The Spirit-filled Christian

If you haven't figured it out by now, the life God calls us to live is impossible: to be pure and holy, to forgive others who have hurt us, to live by faith and not by sight, to die to self daily, and to share the Good News of God's salvation and healing power with our neighbors and the entire world. This is impossible to do in our own strength, but God has given us our Helper, the Holy Spirit, to accomplish all of this and more. Once again, it is all about God!

As we become obedient to the small things He has called us to do, He will begin to let us be a part of greater works He has prepared for us ahead of time. This is when the Christian life truly becomes exciting! Our faith grows as we trust more and more in God's perfect plan for our lives. There are no complicated formulas to learn or difficult exercises to perform to live this kind of life. God has made it simple for us all and He has no favorites.

He does, however, have those who are more intimate with Him. All He requires is for us to surrender completely to Him, to meditate and reflect on His Word, to seek Him with all of our heart, mind, soul, and strength, to pray and to spend time with those of faith in prayer, study, and in confession, and above all else to remain humble. Even though He requires these disciplines and obedience to His Word, He gives us the desires of our heart and helps us to be obedient when we surrender all! It is truly all about Him; He is the author and perfecter of our faith.

Recently, God graciously allowed me to participate in three miracles. I share these with you only to encourage you that God, the Creator of the universe, still uses flawed and unworthy people for great things. But thanks be to God for making me perfect by the blood of Jesus so that I can be used in spite of all of my shortcomings!

Miracle 1: "We have a medical emergency," the flight attendant announced about 25 minutes before landing in Portland. "Are there any doctors or medical professionals onboard?" A few individuals responded immediately, so I remained in my seat and lifted up a prayer: "Lord, if You want to use me in this situation, I am available."

When a flight attendant walked up the aisle, I asked her about the emergency. "Are you a doctor?" she said. Then she told me there was a woman in the rear of the plane who was shaking uncontrollably either from anxiety or a seizure. The medications she was on indicated that she was being treated for a particular illness. I told the flight attendant that if the woman didn't improve within the next couple of minutes, perhaps I could help.

When the commotion didn't subside, I calmly walked to the back of the plane and talked to another flight attendant who said the woman seemed to be getting worse. I saw a middle-aged Chinese woman with her arms and legs shaking dramatically as a woman next to her, a nurse, tried to calm her down. I told the nurse that I was an acupuncturist and that I could do some acupressure on the woman. The nurse agreed, then went with a flight attendant to get a blood pressure cuff.

I sat next to the woman, pressed the acupressure points between her thumb and the index finger, and started praying quietly, "Spirit of fear, leave this woman in the name of Jesus." I continued in prayer, saying, "Thank You, Jesus, for healing this woman. Thank You, Jesus, thank You."

As I prayed, the shaking diminished until it stopped within a minute or two. Meanwhile, the nurse and a couple of flight attendants came rushing back only to see a completely different scene: a calm patient with her eyes closed. As I proceeded to return to my seat, the nurse shouted out, "What did you just do?"

"A little acupressure and prayer," I said quietly and walked back to my seat silently praising the Lord. Furthermore, I gave a brief testimony to several passengers who recognized they had just witnessed a miracle. Praise be to God!

Miracle 2: The next day I got a call from the mother of one of my patients who was in the hospital. Her son, Samuel, was scheduled for a biopsy on his leg (tibia) for a fast-growing tumor that had been diagnosed as an inchondroma a few months prior. The tumor was about the size of a baseball and in a location that was difficult to operate on.

I had seen Samuel for the first time about a month before his biopsy and had offered some herbal and dietary strategies to help bolster his immune system.

That day at Oregon Health Sciences University, the doctor who was going to do the biopsy found no tumor! He said that sometimes mistakes are made with the initial X-rays and/or MRI's, but that was not the case here. The family gave testimony to God's healing power! All that remained of the tumor was a small area of necrotic bone that the doctor was able to scrape away and a residual infection that was treated with antibiotics. Praise be to God!

Miracle 3: This same week, my father-in-law was coming to visit and see my daughter perform in "The Nutcracker." My anxious wife, who had not seen her dad in almost a year after the drama of her parents' divorce, had a lot of deep-seated pain from her dad's choices and was having a hard time holding herself back from scolding him. My only hope for Fereydun was that he would humble himself before the Lord and ask Jesus into his heart and life.

This week being the week of miracles, I had the faith and belief that the Lord could do anything—including opening the eyes of someone whose pride stood in the way. That Sunday morning, December 3, 2006, I entered the guestroom where Fereydun was sleeping and tapped him on the shoulder. "Good morning," he said.

"Baba," I said—that is his nickname—"is it okay if I say a prayer for you?" He agreed, so I began by praying, "Spirit of pride, I command you to leave Fereydun in the name of Jesus." I then prayed that the Lord would reveal Himself to Baba and show him His grace and mercy, which we all need. I then thanked God and let Him know my hopes of seeing Fereydun and his family restored to one another. "Amen," I said, and so did Baba.

That morning at church the service was about religious hypocrites who mislead people by not sharing the truth that only Jesus can heal and restore souls and lives by what He accomplished on the cross. All we have to do is to believe in Him and receive Him as our Lord and Master. Even though Fereydun had heard this message before, He seemed to be acknowledging what he heard. After the service, while in the car with him and my son, I could not hold back asking him, "Baba, I know this is a private question for you, but I am going to ask it anyway. What is holding you back from asking the Lord into your heart?"

"Shaun, like you said, this is a very private matter to me, but when your pastor Phil spoke today, I felt as if he was speaking directly to me. I never have wanted to be a hypocrite myself, and I have never made this decision before because I did not feel that God was real to me. But today, I asked the Lord into my heart. I don't know what that all means and I want to take it at my own pace, but I did take my decision very seriously."

Praise be to the God of miracles! I hope this seed falls into good soil and bears fruit (see Matthew 13).

Where Are You?

No matter where you find yourself on the mountain today, reflect on the God stories in your life—on His love story in the Bible and in the lives of those He has placed in your life. Remember that God can take any ugly situation and turn it into something beautiful in time. Yes, it may take time, patience, and a lot of prayer, but remember the fact that God is working out everything for the good of those who love Him and obey His commands.

Do you want to live the Spirit-filled life? There are plenty of compromised Christians who are living out lukewarm lives for God and have been put on the bench, never truly being used by God. I hope and pray that you want all that God has in store for those who love Him and follow His ways.

It all starts with your willingness to surrender all! Your dreams, your hopes, your pains, your relationships, your finances, your health, and most importantly your heart and mind.

Then pray daily, *Lord, not my will but Thy will be done. Mold me, shape me, and change me into the person You want me to be.* Spend time in His Word, in prayer, and in worship daily. Trust me—no, trust God and His Word—you will not be disappointed at who you become and how your life begins to form into something you could not have dreamed of yourself. God is good!

CHAPTER 3
Thriving in Your Mind (and Heart)

3.1 Time to De-weed

Your mind and your emotions are the chief battlefields for your peace. Jealousy, envy, greed, worry, fear, anger, resentment, depression, guilt, and shame—these are some of the thoughts and feelings that rob us of peace and drive many to the counselor's office. And of course counseling is one of the better places to end up. Many of these destructive thoughts and feelings can send people to the hospital for cancer, stroke, or heart attack, or to prison for irrational criminal acts. Most commonly, you end up in autopilot mode, enduring a miserable existence.

In order to thrive in your mind and emotions—*i.e.,* to have peace, hope, and joy—you must untangle yourself from these worldly traps. The Bible has plenty to say on this subject. Just like the weeds in a garden need to be pulled on a regular basis, your negative thoughts must be intentionally removed—*and replaced with holy thoughts.* This is where God's sovereignty and our responsibility meet head on, and where many people give up in failure. They settle for an average life instead of seizing the more abundant life that God calls us to.

If you want to experience God's truths and promises to the

fullest extent, you must fully commit to this process! Many of God's promises and covenants with His people throughout the ages are conditional on doing what He commands. As you will see throughout this chapter, if you are truly committed to God and His will, He will help you with every step. The key, as you will discover, is keeping your focus on God, denying yourself, and getting to know Jesus intimately by spending time with Him. This is the only way that your head knowledge will begin to translate into your heart and soul reality.

Perception Is Reality (or Is It?)

We all have our own thought systems based on our childhood experiences, traumas in our lives, things we have been taught and have read about, and ideas we have incorporated into our minds. The truth is that many of them could be false. After coming to know God personally, we need to examine our beliefs and be renewed in our thinking. This new way of thinking begins with awakening to the truth about who God is, understanding and applying His Word, and communicating with Him as we saw in Chapter 2. Awakening leads us to revolutionary, earth-shaking truths. The next step is to begin the process of being "awake" every moment, to apply this knowledge of God to every area of our lives. We bring our minds and our entire way of thinking in line with what has happened to us spiritually.

To keep these truths tucked away in a corner of the mind, separated from everyday life, is the same as denying that they are true. Can we really claim that we believe in the existence of a Creator, who rules the universe, if we don't care what He thinks about the decisions we are about to make? Our moment-to-moment thinking and our daily decisions and behavior reveal our true beliefs. If we claim to believe in a real, vital, personal, living God, we must see every part of life in the light of this truth.

This new way of thinking gives us a brand-new, spectacularly different view of life—one so different that it enables us to thrive spiritually, mentally, and emotionally, regardless of our circumstances and challenges. There is a direct physiological connection of a sound mind and peaceful spirit on our physical well-being, which I will expand on in Chapter 4. We now have the potential, as never before, to live with both courage and serenity, to grow, laugh, love and be loved. To have peace, joy, patience, and hope in and through our circumstances. Will this be an easy process? Absolutely not! Jesus said, *"If anyone would come after me, he must deny himself and take up his cross and follow me. For whoever wants to save his life will lose it, but whoever loses his life for me will find it."*[54] The ugly ego has to be put to rest daily if we are truly to grow and thrive.

In the area of our personal growth, we will find that mysterious interplay between our responsibility and God's sovereign power playing out. We grow as we cooperate with God and obey Him. Yet, at the same time, He may be "growing" us and causing us to cooperate with Him. He will challenge us, mold us, and even break us in order to shape us into the person He always wanted us to be. We seem to have a choice: to grudgingly give as little of ourselves to Him as possible, rebelling and complaining as we go, or reaching up to Him with open, trusting arms. The first of these paths is unrewarding, unpleasant, and outright painful. The other, even when life brings grief and challenges, is the path of profound peace and heart-thrilling joy.

This new way of thinking is described in full in God's Word. Other than prayer, nothing is more important than reading the Bible. It is the starting place of the believer's life. His Word is His love letter to us and contains His instructions for life. It has a depth and complexity greater than any book ever written, yet its messages are simple and clear enough for the least educated people to understand, if God opens up their hearts and minds. As Psalm 119 says, *"Your word is a lamp to my feet and a light for my path."*[55]

The most important message of God's Word is who God is, who we are, and how to have an authentic, intimate, loving

---

[54] Matthew 16:24-25
[55] Verse 105

relationship with God, now and for eternity. But within its pages you'll also discover this life-changing way of thinking. God provides us with the gift of His perspective on all aspects of life, including relationships, money, the meaning of life, how to raise children, how to worship, what to do about anger, how to have a happy marriage, the purpose of suffering, and how to avoid temptations. God's Word also counsels us about sin, which may at times appear attractive, fun, or exciting, but the consequences are dire. Sin separates you from God and leaves you vulnerable to your enemy, satan. When you have a relationship with God, He gives you the power of His Holy Spirit to resist temptation and to overcome sin.

Much of the wisdom in God's Word relates directly and dramatically to the mind-body-spirit connection that I see operating in the lives of the people I know and treat. Stress, in particular, is a significant factor in wellness and disease prevention, as we'll see in more detail in Chapter 4, and nothing addresses the root causes of stress in a more effective, permanent, and meaningful way than believing, understanding, and living by God's Word.

In Chapter 2, understanding and applying the Serenity Prayer summed up how to thrive spiritually. In this chapter we'll discuss the Lord's Prayer. When understood and applied, this prayer that the Lord Himself taught to His disciples sums up how to thrive in our minds and hearts. We will be examining aspects of this prayer throughout this chapter.

Our Father which art in heaven, hallowed be thy name. Thy kingdom come, thy will be done in earth, as it is in heaven. Give us this day our daily bread. And forgive us our debts, as we forgive our debtors. And lead us not into temptation, but deliver us from evil: For thine is the kingdom, and the power, and the glory, for ever. Amen.[56]

This simple, humble prayer is packed with meaningful phrases.

---

[56] Matthew 6:9-13 King James Version

It establishes first who God is: Father, Hallowed (Holy) One, and King. He wants us to address Him as Father because just like a human father He wants to be in a close, loving relationship with us. As our Father, He sympathizes with us, wants to help, protect, and teach us, and wants us to turn out well. He won't deny us anything good. He will discipline us for our own good. He is also our King. Because He is the all-powerful King, He is able to help us in any situation. Describing Him also reaffirms who *we* are: He is the Father, I am His child. He is holy; I am not, except through Jesus. He is King, I am His subject. The Lord's Prayer then asks for God's will to be done, rather than ours. It asks God to give us our "daily bread." This may include food, but more importantly it is God and His Word alone that will truly satisfy. We need this spiritual food "daily"! The prayer is asking for what we need today, not tomorrow. God wants us to walk hand in hand with Him through each day, as His children, totally trusting and dependent on Him. Then, the prayer asks for forgiveness and acknowledges our responsibility to forgive others, just as God has forgiven us. Finally, the prayer asks for protection from temptation and evil and once again acknowledges His power and glory now and for eternity.

This prayer doesn't necessarily contain the thoughts we would come up with on our own, without God's influence, does it? Learning from this prayer involves the necessary process of lining up our wills with God's will, of modeling our hearts after God's heart. God does not make it complicated! All we have to do is focus on Him personally and die to our ego daily. Then we can have a mind at peace and a heart free from anxiety.

3.2 A Mind and Heart at Peace

A positive mental attitude is essential for anyone who wants to be truly healthy, both emotionally and physically. *"A heart at peace gives life to the body."*[57] Many of us have negative tape

---

[57] Proverbs 14:30

recordings stored in our heads, and we're constantly replaying messages that focus on our unworthiness, our failures, our problems, our imperfections, our past wrongdoings. These messages make life miserable. They predispose us for future failures, and they compel us to perceive normal life events as threatening and stressful. In the Victim and Controller stages of ego, we may follow the instructions of self-help books and strive to be upbeat and optimistic, to give ourselves only healthy messages, and to use positive affirmations and visualizations. No doubt it is true that an optimistic, positive-thinking person will generally be happier, healthier, and enjoy life more than someone who is pessimistic, self-destructive, and depressed. But deep inside our hearts, we know that a positive attitude only goes so far in helping us. Why? Because only the Word of God—and its truths and promises—will never fail us. God is very real; He does not need for anyone to be in the business of hypnosis, brainwashing, or self-deception.

True, deep, lasting inner peace settles in as we begin to eat, breathe, and become dependent on absolute truth, as we sink roots into ground that can never be shaken, as we stand firm on solid rock. This solid rock is God Himself and His unchanging, absolutely dependable truths. His words are reality. We can trust them completely and fearlessly base our lives on them. The more we turn to these truths, found in His Word, and grasp their meaning, memorize them, meditate on them, and make them part of our being, the happier and more at peace we will be.

1. We can be at peace with God. You'll find the word "peace" more than 250 times in the Bible; God is the *"God of Peace."*[58] In the book of Isaiah, Jesus is called the *"Prince of Peace."*[59] He didn't come to bring peace to this earth, but peace between God and the human race—to everyone who enters into a relationship with Him. This isn't some sort of abstract, symbolic peace. It is real. We were at war with God, rejecting what He said reality is and rejecting what He told us to do. We denied who He

---

[58] Romans 15:33; 2 Corinthians 13:11; Philippians 4:9; Hebrews 13:20
[59] Isaiah 9:6

is, and some of us even denied that He exists at all. When we take the steps that are spelled out in Chapter 2, we are, in effect, asking Jesus to wave a white flag for us, signaling that we surrender. We can now be at peace with God. He is on our side, permanently. In fact, we now can be at peace for eternity. This state of peace is so dramatically different from our old situation that, unless we continue to try to wrestle God for control, it can permeate every part of us. When you made the decision to believe in Jesus, you were fully accepted by God, fully forgiven, righteous and holy in His sight, and deeply loved by Him.

For God was pleased to have all his fullness dwell in him [Jesus], and through him to reconcile to himself all things, whether things on earth or things in heaven, by making peace through his blood, shed on the cross. Once you were alienated from God and were enemies in your minds because of your evil behavior. But now he has reconciled you by Christ's physical body through death to present you holy in his sight, without blemish and free from accusation—if you continue in your faith, established and firm, not moved from the hope held out in the gospel.[60]

It is an amazing feeling to know that we have peace with God. Wherever we go in this life, He will, in effect, be standing there with us: protecting, leading, teaching, and helping. We no longer have to be anxious about what will happen to us when we die. In fact, we no longer have to be anxious about anything.

2. We can be at peace about life's events. When we have a relationship with God, we begin to understand that He is completely in control and that He uses everything in our lives for our ultimate good. *"And we know that in all things God works for the good of those who love him."*[61] As we go through life, we will be amazed by the way He shows us grace and mercy, and works things out for us. But the words in this verse have a deeper

---

[60] Colossians 1:19-23
[61] Romans 8:28

meaning. In the stages of ego, "good" might be defined as winning the lottery, having an easy life, being popular, having power, and getting our way. In the awakened state, however, we realize that "good" means becoming more like Jesus and serving and glorifying God. All of the blessings that God pours out on us are simply a side effect of seeking first the kingdom of God and His righteousness. Our lives are given purpose and meaning. Nothing we do will be wasted. He will use our hard work, talents, and personalities; He will also use our failures, defects, loneliness, and suffering. This knowledge can completely alter our perception of life's events, even the ones that are stressful. Every experience in life can become an opportunity to learn, to serve God, to offer up our pain as a gift to Him, to sacrifice ourselves for people around us, to encourage others or lead them to Jesus.

This is not an excuse to deliberately disobey Him, thinking, "Oh, I can do what I want and He'll turn it into something good." On the contrary, the Bible says that we reap what we sow and that He disciplines those He loves. But if we honestly want to please Him and come to Him confessing our wrongdoings, He is eager to cover over our sins and bless us. *"Great peaces have they who love your law, and nothing can make them stumble."*[62]

On the night Jesus was betrayed by Judas, before He was arrested, He had a long talk with His disciples, explaining many things to them. He then said something that is just as true for us today as it was for the men gathered around Him that night:

"I have told you these things, so that in me you may have peace. In this world you will have trouble. But take heart! I have overcome the world."[63]

3. We can be at peace about the future. The future doesn't belong to us. It belongs to God. In the past, we all put ourselves on the throne and were our own gods. Our emotions were considered sacred, in a way. "This is the way I feel! I can't help how I feel!

---

[62] Psalm 119:165
[63] John 16:33

You can't tell me that my feelings are wrong!" God sees emotions in a different light. He actually commands us not to worry. *"Don't worry about anything; instead, pray about everything. Tell God what you need, and thank him for all he has done. If you do this, you will experience God's peace, which is far more wonderful than the human mind can understand. His peace will guard your hearts and minds as you live in Christ Jesus."*[64]

When God commands us to do something and we don't do it, that is sin. Worry is a sin that He takes seriously. Why? Because at its core is a disbelief and distrust of Him. Most of us will struggle with this sin our entire lives, but we must not give in and accept it as normal. Each time you have a worried thought, confess it to God immediately. See it for what it is: lack of faith in His ability to direct the course of your life according to His will. He responds lovingly and tenderly to us when we come to Him. *"Cast all your anxiety on him because he cares for you."*[65] Instead of being at the mercy of every fleeting emotion, God empowers us to base our thought lives on reality: the reality that He is completely faithful and trustworthy. I make it a conscious choice to give the Lord all my troubles as well as "my" successes and glory.

Most of what we worry about displays that our priorities are confused. Are you worried more about money or about obeying God? Are you fretting over what your employer thinks of you or are you deeply concerned about what God thinks of your current job? Which is a greater concern to you: getting everything done on your list of things to do, or serving God today and doing what is on His list? Worry, as most of us have come to realize, accomplishes nothing. After all, as Jesus said, *"Do not worry about your life, what you will eat or drink; or about your body, what you will wear.... Who of you by worrying can add a single hour to his life? But seek first his kingdom and his righteousness, and all these things will be given to you as well. Therefore, do not worry about tomorrow, for tomorrow will worry about itself. Each day*

---

[64] Philippians 4:6-7 New Living Translation
[65] 1 Peter 5:7

has enough trouble of its own. "[66]

Seek God first; seek what He wants from you each day. The more we trust in Him and see Him as truly God, the less we will worry, and the more peace we will have. *"I will lie down and sleep in peace, for you alone, O LORD, make me dwell in safety."*[67]

4. We can be at peace with other people. When we become believers, we accept an entirely different reality about people. We realize that we have a relationship with God not because we're special in any way but simply because of what Jesus did for us. As we look around, we begin to see that everyone falls into two groups. There are the people, like us, who are now forgiven sinners, undeserving of a relationship with God, but who, because of His grace and mercy, are now His children. Then there are the people who don't know God, who need His love and forgiveness. We have no basis on which to look down on anyone. (In fact, God asks more of us. He set us free from slavery to wrongdoing and sin. We have a choice, and the help we need to make the right choice.) Both groups contain people like us, who make mistakes, who have social blind spots, who are deliberately selfish at times, who offend others, consciously or not. Both groups need compassion, the truth spoken in love, a helping (but not enabling) hand. God loved us when we hated Him, even if, in your case perhaps, the hatred took the form of just ignoring Him. He loved us and made the ultimate sacrifice. It is on the basis of what He did for us that we determine how to act toward other people, rather than on the basis of how they act toward us: to love them when they don't deserve it. This is a radically new way for most of us to think.

However, we aren't just supposed to be tolerant and accepting. We still see that some things are plainly wrong and others plainly right in God's eyes. We must not ever help someone to continue in sin. We need discernment so that we can determine who can provide us with wise counsel, who would be a trusted friend, who would make a good role model, who fulfills God's criteria for

---

[66] Matthew 6:25, 27, 33, 34
[67] Psalm 4:8

leadership in the church, who is suitable for marriage, and so forth. Some people should only be loved from a distance for our own safety. But, generally speaking, seeing people through God's eyes will give us the opportunity, as never before, to be at peace with them.

We also can be at peace with other people because we are in obedience to God. *"When a man's ways are pleasing to the LORD, he makes even his enemies live at peace with him."*[68] *"Do not repay anyone evil for evil. Be careful to do what is right in the eyes of everybody. If it is possible, as far as it depends on you, live at peace with everyone."*[69] This doesn't mean we are conformists; in fact, God's Word cautions us against conforming to the ways of this world. Instead, we are to be yielding, gentle, humble, patient people, seeking not to offend anyone for selfish reasons. Because this goes against the basic nature of most of us, we will need God's help and much prayer.

5. We can be at peace with ourselves. Fairly recently, a philosophy has developed in our culture that people have been eager to believe. This philosophy says that we need to learn to love ourselves. Psychologists talk about it, movie stars name it as their highest goal, and talk show hosts discuss it endlessly as if it is truth from on high. Despite the fact that no one seems to have achieved it in any satisfying or long-lasting way, most people in our culture are beginning to believe that it is what life is all about. God predicted this development 2,000 years ago. *"But mark this: There will be terrible times in the last days. People will be lovers of themselves...."*[70] Jesus called His followers to exactly the opposite behavior. *"If anyone would come after me,"* He said, *"he must deny himself and take up his cross daily and follow me."*[71]

Virtually everyone who isn't mentally ill already loves himself to the extent necessary for a good life. As discussed in Chapter 1, we love ourselves enough to provide food, clothing, shelter, and

---

[68] Proverbs 16:7
[69] Romans 12:17-18
[70] 2 Timothy 3:1-2
[71] Luke 9:23

medicine. We try to avoid physical pain and we hope for good experiences and don't think, "Gee, I wish something bad would happen to me." If each of us wanted these things as much for our neighbors as for ourselves, the world would be in spectacularly better shape. But any self-love beyond that which is needed for self-preservation just won't work. Why? Because we weren't created to first love ourselves. We have been created to love God first and above all else. Attempts to focus on loving ourselves and building self-esteem backfire. It simply fuels our ego and ultimately separates us from God.

When we strive for self-esteem, we have a problem. We know our defects. We know that we aren't worthy of honor and esteem. We hope that no one else will notice. As you go through the day interacting with people, would you like them all to hear the thoughts going through your mind? Would you like them to know what tempts you, the exaggerations you have spoken, the false humility in your words, the judgmental thoughts you've had, or how often you are motivated by a desire for the approval of others? If we somehow have a high view of ourselves, it is fragile. An encounter with the Bible, our mother, spouse, sibling, child, aunt, tax accountant, job interviewer, a party, a golf game, a bathroom scale, or the doctor could bring us toppling down from our self-made throne in a matter of minutes. We know in our hearts that we aren't worthy of God's love. And we are right. We have value because God loves us, not the other way around.

When we long for the ability to love ourselves, we are seeking something that will not fix what is broken in us. What we are usually attempting to cure with self-love is all the negative self-talk in our heads. But the cure for that isn't playing an imaginary tape that says, "I'm great! I'm worthy of love!" This doesn't satisfy us. The cure is to turn our focus away from ourselves toward God.

We need to recognize that our thought lives are a place of spiritual warfare. God wants us to focus on Him, on loving Him and living for Him. Fighting against this are three influences: the ego, the world's philosophies and lusts, and the force of evil. The ego wants us to live for ourselves, not God. The world, too, promotes a selfish life, grabbing as much as we can of what it offers, even if it means losing what heaven offers. The force of evil (which many of us are uncomfortable acknowledging even exists) wants us to live for anything but God.

What are the tools of these three influences that war against our souls? Thoughts in our minds that threaten to defeat us, such as confusion, doubt, fear, envy, feelings of condemnation, pride, vanity, boredom, deception, busyness. The lusting of our eyes that appeals to our desire for possessions and preys on feelings of inferiority. And people who, in a manner of speaking, know where our "buttons" are and how to push them. When you enter into a relationship with the living God, you can expect distractions to keep you from fully devoting yourself to Him, temptations to sway you just a little bit off the path, and deceptions to cause you to doubt what God has said in His Word.

Satan is called *"the accuser."*[72] While it is true that God makes us aware of our wrongdoing, His response is to ask us to turn away from our misbehavior and wrong attitudes (repent), draw close to Him, receive His forgiveness, and be in loving fellowship with Him. In contrast, satan sends messages that put us down. "I'm a terrible person," "I can never change," "I'm ugly," and "I hate myself" are not thoughts from God; they are accusations and condemnations. They cause misery and self-hatred. But even hating ourselves keeps our focus on ourselves, where it doesn't belong.

How can we win this battle?

First, depend on God. Controlling the thought life and having peace is a lifelong struggle for nearly everyone and really only happens when we depend fully on God. Once we have entered into a relationship with Him, He begins to remake us, including our thought life, if we continually turn to Him. The Bible says, *"You were taught, with regard to your former way of life, to put off your old self, which is being corrupted by its deceitful desires; to be made new in the attitude of your minds; and to put on the new self, created to be like God in true righteousness and holiness."*[73]

---

[72] Revelation 12:10
[73] Ephesians 4:22-24

Bring every miserable thought to Him, even if you need to do it 200 times a day. "Lord, take this worry from me. Help me trust You." "Lord, help me to feel how much You love me." "Lord, help me to understand that You have fully forgiven me and have wiped me completely clean." "Lord, help me to grab hold of the joy that You offer." "Lord, help me to obey You, to surrender to You completely in this." "Lord, help me to let go of the past."

Second, discard the illusions about who you are without Jesus Christ. Denial of our natural state will not help us, but only hinder our ability to recognize sin in our lives and confess it. Refusal to accept this is often a telltale sign that we think we are partially responsible for our salvation, that we were somehow worthy of salvation. Let's look at what God has to say:

To some who were confident of their own righteousness and looked down on everybody else, Jesus told this parable: "Two men went up to the temple to pray, one a Pharisee [Pharisees were considered to be the most religious and righteous people of that day and culture] and the other a tax collector. The Pharisee stood up and prayed about himself: 'God, I thank you that I am not like other men—robbers, evildoers, adulterers—or even like this tax collector. I fast twice a week and give a tenth of all I get.' But the tax collector stood at a distance. He would not even look up to heaven, but beat his breast and said, 'God, have mercy on me, a sinner.' I tell you that this man, rather than the other, went home justified before God. For everyone who exalts himself will be humbled, and he who humbles himself will be exalted."[74]

During your daily prayer and reading of God's Word, learn to examine your heart in His presence. Reading His Word presents you with a mirror. You can see yourself in what you are reading. Ask Him to reveal what needs to change inside of you.

Do not merely listen to the word, and so deceive yourselves. Do what it says. Anyone who listens to the word but does not do

---

[74] Luke 18:9-14

what it says is like a man who looks at his face in a mirror and, after looking at himself, goes away and immediately forgets what he looks like. But the man who looks intently into the perfect law that gives freedom, and continues to do this, not forgetting what he has heard, but doing it—he will be blessed in what he does.[75]

Confess that, yes, these things need to change. Pray for God's help. Recognize that carrying guilt merely keeps you from going to God for forgiveness and cleansing. Don't slip back into self-condemnation, which robs you of the joy that is available to you in Christ. Confession, repentance, and obedience sound terrible to people living in the stages of ego, but they are words of freedom and peace to those who are awakened.

Third, embrace your new identity in Christ. *"Therefore, if anyone is in Christ, he is a new creation; the old has gone, the new has come!"*[76] There is a lot of good news! To start with, God has set you free from slavery to your own wrongdoing. He chose you before the creation of the world. Jesus lives in your heart through faith. (Not just in the way that we say a deceased loved one is still "alive" in our hearts. Jesus actually is alive in heaven, after rising from the dead, and actively works in our hearts through His Holy Spirit.) He empowers you to mature spiritually, to act rightly, to reject sin, and to really love people. You have all the righteousness of Jesus credited to your account. God will *"take great delight in you, he will quiet you with his love, he will rejoice over you with singing."*[77] You have a unique role to play for Him here on earth that no one else can fulfill. You are a loved child of God, precious in His sight. As someone who has a real relationship with the living God, you can enter into His presence with confidence and speak to Him and lay your requests before Him. You are now an heir of the kingdom of heaven, and you will live forever in God's presence. This is the God esteem that I mentioned in Chapter 1. How could your esteem not be affected by

---

[75] James 1:22-25
[76] 2 Corinthians 5:17
[77] Zephaniah 3:17

the fact that He sent His Son to die for you on the cross at Calvary, adopting you into His heavenly family, a royal priesthood!

These are reasons for joy, thanksgiving, and peace! These are the things to remember when you are tempted to play back those negative tapes in your mind.

3.3 Our Daily Bread

Immerse your mind in the things that are of God:

- Before you get out of bed in the morning, share your first thoughts with God, thanking Him for the day ahead, reaffirming that you want to honor, trust, and obey Him, and asking Him to guide your behavior, words, and thoughts that day.
- Join a fellowship of believers who uncompromisingly follow God's Word and joyfully worship Him. Meet with them at least once a week.
- Read the Bible daily. Ask God to show you what He wants you to notice as you read. Reflect on what you've read. You may find it supportive to join a Bible study to help answer questions and to hear others share their faith. I like to read at least a proverb and a psalm daily.
- Set aside time to pray, perhaps after you've done your daily reading. Submit your requests to God, for yourself and for other people. Prayer also includes expressing gratitude, listening, praise, and worship. Consider keeping a list of prayer requests in a notebook. Review it occasionally to see how God has answered them. Review your interactions with people throughout the day, your thoughts and feelings about them, and confess each thing, big or small, that grieves God. This daily confession will keep your conscience clear and bring you the peace that comes from God's forgiveness. This honesty before God also helps you to grow spiritually.

- Have a regular time for family worship. Read a passage from God's Word and briefly discuss it. Sing a song together or pray together.
- Ask God to open your eyes to people around you who are suffering. Look for ways to help them and to share God's love with them.
- Listen to music that praises God. Introduce your children to this music and sing it together.
- Read the life stories of well-known believers.

Meditate on God's Word. We are instructed to *"Set your minds on things above, not on earthly things."*[78] God also tells us: *"whatever is true, whatever is noble, whatever is right, whatever is pure, whatever is lovely, whatever is admirable—if anything is excellent or praiseworthy—think about such things."*[79] The surest way to obey these commands is to meditate on God's Word.

Meditation is misunderstood. Many people associate meditation with a spiritual practice of Eastern religions that has been adopted by Western and "alternative" medicine as a relaxation technique. But, from God's point of view, this kind of meditation isn't a true spiritual practice. True spirituality always relates directly to the living God. Without Him, there is no spirituality, there is no spirit, there is only the ego.

In contrast, what the Bible calls meditation focuses on God and His Word. It involves contemplation, reflection, memorization, and listening. Meditation goes hand in hand with prayer. It is the process by which we find the connection between God's Word and our lives. Meditating on God's Word will lead to quietness of heart and life, even if you do it on the bus, in traffic, on a walk, or while you eat. God's Word describes meditation in a variety of settings:

In your anger do not sin; when you are on your beds, search your hearts and be silent.[80]

---

[78] Colossians 3:2
[79] Philippians 4:8
[80] Psalm 4:4

He went out to the field one evening to meditate.[81]

Within your temple, O God, we meditate on your unfailing love.[82]

As you review these examples of meditation found in God's Word, consider how this is not merely an intellectual activity. Meditation is part of an intimate relationship with the living God, an opportunity for delight, communication, and healing. He instructs and corrects us, encourages and guides us, and gives us hope.

I rise before dawn and cry for help; I have put my hope in your word. My eyes stay open through the watches of the night, that I may meditate on your promises.[83]

I remember the days of long ago; I meditate on all your works and consider what your hands have done. I spread out my hands to you; my soul thirsts for you like a parched land.[84]

When your words came, I ate them; they were my joy and my heart's delight, for I bear your name, O LORD God Almighty.[85]

All Scripture is God-breathed and is useful for teaching, rebuking, correcting and training in righteousness."[86]

For everything that was written in the past was written to teach us, so that through endurance and the encouragement of the Scriptures we might have hope.[87]

---

[81] Genesis 24:63
[82] Psalm 48:9
[83] Psalm 119:147-148
[84] Psalm 143:5-6
[85] Jeremiah 15:16
[86] 2 Timothy 3:16
[87] Romans 15:4

Meditate on God's characteristics—for example, He is faithful, patient, merciful, holy, righteous, all knowing, just, and loving. Meditate on the amazing things He has done throughout history, in your life, and in the lives of your friends. What has God done this day or week in your life? Meditate on what He has created, and what that reveals about Him. An excellent time to meditate on God's Word or God Himself is while you are walking, or perhaps after you've used the relaxation methods described in the thriving physically chapter. Meditate on selected verses. For example, James 3:13-18 discusses earthly versus heavenly wisdom. You might write these verses on an index card, take it with you on a walk, and think about their implications. As you read any passage in God's Word, ask yourself: What does this tell me about Jesus, His Father, or His Holy Spirit? How does this passage apply to me?

Live in the present moment. How much of your time do you spend fantasizing about the future, worrying, planning but not taking action, longing for what you don't have? Or how often are you reliving painful moments from the past, caused by your own wrongdoings or by offenses committed against you? Perhaps the pain comes from shame, or maybe you're chained to memories of terrible things inflicted on you in your childhood.

Learn to turn all of these past and future-oriented thoughts over to God. Each time you catch yourself thinking in these patterns, stop and ask God to help you focus on something He would like you to think about. Take these thoughts of the past and future, no matter how deep and painful the cause may be, and lay them at the foot of the cross. If it takes you a hundred times, do it a hundred times. God wants you to let go of them. He wants to set you free from the past, and He wants you to see that the future is in His hands, not yours. Let Him carry the burden. Learning from your past mistakes and not repeating them is a useful exercise, and following the dreams that the Lord has implanted in your heart brings joy and fulfillment. When we become wrapped up in the past or fantasize about the future, however, we miss the gift of the present moment. There are some things we should look forward to: seeing an old friend, going on a vacation, Sunday worship, and the glorious day we will see our Savior face to face and our loved ones in heaven. Until that time, we must live the victorious life, walking and communing with our Creator and His (our) family on a daily basis!

Recognize the source of your thoughts. God does convict us of sin; His Holy Spirit constantly points out our disobedient thoughts and actions so we can confess them to Him and receive forgiveness. But confusion, worry, anxiety, condemnation, fear, envy, pride, resentment, and defensiveness are not from God. If you catch yourself thinking this way, put on the brakes immediately and turn to God.

Memorize Scripture. As you read the Bible, underline any verse that especially speaks to your heart. Write it down on an index card and review it throughout the day—while you're waiting in line, waiting in traffic, taking a walk, doing the dishes. Learn the reference to chapter and verse at the same time. Say it out loud. Review everything that you've memorized each week. Choose verses that encourage you, that will help you tell people about God, or that will help you remember what is right. This is critical for the renewing of your mind. Remember, garbage in, garbage out; God's truths and promises, however, bear beautiful fruit over time.

If you have not done so already, take the time right now to write down five Bible verses on separate index cards that you will begin to commit to memory. Many of the verses already quoted in this chapter, and the ones that follow, have helped countless individuals begin to renew their minds. Add to your collection of memory verses—you will not be disappointed that you took this effort. God's Word never fails to accomplish its purpose; it always bears fruit! Review your memory verses daily until they are firmly implanted in your consciousness and subconsciousness, and begin to overflow from your soul.

"For I know the plans I have for you," declares the LORD, "plans to prosper you and not to harm you, plans to give you

hope and a future."[88]

"Fear not, for I have redeemed you; I have summoned you by name; you are mine. When you pass through the waters, I will be with you; and when you pass through the rivers, they will not sweep over you."[89]

If we confess our sins, he is faithful and just and will forgive us our sins and purify us from all unrighteousness.[90]

Everyone should be quick to listen, slow to speak and slow to become angry, for man's anger does not bring about the righteous life that God desires.[91]

And my God will meet all your needs according to his glorious riches in Christ Jesus."[92]

Rejoice in the Lord always. I will say it again: Rejoice![93]

Therefore confess your sins to each other and pray for each other so that you may be healed. The prayer of a righteous man is powerful and effective.[94]

Blessed is the man who fears the LORD, who finds great delight in his commands. His children will be mighty in the land; the generation of the upright will be blessed. Wealth and riches are in his house, and his righteousness endures forever.[95]

You may find the following portion of Scripture from the Old

---

[88] Jeremiah 29:11
[89] Isaiah 43:1-2
[90] 1 John 1:9
[91] James 1:19-20
[92] Philippians 4:19
[93] Philippians 4:4
[94] James 5:16
[95] Psalm 112:1-3

Testament a bit too long to memorize, but, like the psalm above, these verses show God's desire to bless us. We're also reminded that God's promises have some conditions. This covenant was with God's chosen people, the newly formed nation of Israel, but the principles apply to every believer:

If you listen to these regulations and obey them faithfully, the LORD your God will keep his covenant of unfailing love with you, as he solemnly promised your ancestors. He will love you and bless you and make you into a great nation. He will give you many children and give fertility to your land and your animals. When you arrive in the land he swore to give your ancestors, you will have large crops of grain, grapes, and olives, and great herds of cattle, sheep, and goats. You will be blessed above all nations of the earth. None of your men or women will be childless, and all your livestock will bear young. And the LORD will protect you from all sickness. He will not let you suffer from the terrible diseases you knew in Egypt, but he will bring them all on your enemies.[96]

Before you get too excited and confident that you are somehow achieving this kind of covenant relationship with God or that you can in the future, think again. All of the great saints of the Old Testament and New Testament broke the conditions of God's covenants by their sins. You and I are no different. Do not be like Job who asked the question or at least implied, "What did I do to deserve all of this?" None of us deserves God's love, grace, mercy, protection, or promises. The New and Everlasting Covenant is found only in the sacrificial death of Jesus. This is the one-sided equation of God's undeserved grace and mercy at Christ's expense.

Our part in the equation is simply to confess our sins and turn to God. Don't even think that you or I have the ability to confess our sins and repent without God's help. It is simply all about Him!

Here are five questions for you and your group to discuss to see if you are on track:

---

[96] Deuteronomy 7:12-15

1. Today have you submitted all your dreams, hopes, plans, and anxieties and worries to your Creator? Can you honestly say, "Thy will be done in my life"?

2. Are there any thoughts that need de-weeding today? Remember, your thought life is the chief battlefield for your peace, so it's likely that you'll struggle in this area at times if not daily. Therefore it's critical that you examine your thought life daily!

3. What Scripture verses are important today for the renewing of your mind? Do you have them memorized? Are they beginning to move from your mind into your heart (*i.e.*, they're not just head knowledge)?

4. What blessings has God done in your life recently? Share one of them with your group or a close friend to offer encouragement.

5. Are there any sins that you need to confess today? Remember, repentance is turning in the opposite direction of your error in thought or action.

3.4 Thy Will Be Done

The Lord's Prayer proclaims, ***"Thy will be done on earth as it is in heaven."*** Knowing God's will is not as complicated as we sometimes make it out to be. It is essentially a life characterized by intimate relationships, holiness, order, and worship. Until the return of Jesus Christ and the descent of the heavenly Jerusalem to earth, we are called to live out this calling by the power of the Holy Spirit. Being in the center of God's will is the safest and most fulfilling place to be!

Here are 12 principles/commands you can be sure are God's will for your life:

1. The Principle of Stewardship
Take care of what God has given you

Ultimately, everything belongs to God, who has charged us with the responsibility of caring for what He has created: the earth, nature, our families, our special gifts and abilities, our money, and even our bodies. We were put on earth to help accomplish God's purposes. *"For we are God's workmanship, created in Christ Jesus to do good works, which God prepared in advance for us to do."*[97] The word translated "workmanship" has several meanings in Greek (the language in which the New Testament was originally written), one of which is a "work of art." Human beings are indeed a great work of art, and while we will eventually shed our bodies for our new heavenly ones, for the time being your body is your dwelling place. In fact, if we have a relationship with the living God, His Holy Spirit lives in us. *"Do you not know that your body is a temple of the Holy Spirit, who is in you, whom you have received from God."*[98] Our greatest motivation for taking care of ourselves, each other, and our planet properly should be because God created us and entrusted us with the care of all things.

2. The Principle of Forgiveness
Forgive others as God has forgiven you

The "Our Father" prayer says, *"Forgive us of our trespasses as we forgive those who trespass against us."* Forgiveness is something God requires in order for us to be forgiven of our habitual sin. This is not referring to salvation, which has been paid once and for all by the blood of Christ. This is referring to our need for continual repentance and our need to acknowledge fully that God has forgiven us of all of our sins—past, present, and future—when we repent. Do we deserve this kind of forgiveness? Absolutely not! That is why God requires us to forgive others as

---

[97] Ephesians 2:10
[98] 1 Corinthians 6:19

we recognize the grace and mercy He has given us. God's grace primarily refers to the undeserved favor He shows to those who have a relationship with Him, when He pays the penalty for our unrighteousness, grants us forgiveness, and prepares a home in heaven for us. But He also shows us grace here and now. He knows that we aren't perfect, that we have many frailties. He has compassion for us and not only is pleased to help us but actually wants us to depend on Him.

If grace is getting what we don't deserve, mercy is not getting what we do deserve. Even after you become a believer, you still have your sinful nature. Sanctification is the process in which God begins to make us holy, begins conforming us to the image of His Son, and sets us apart for His holy purposes. When we sin, we deserve the due punishment or consequences of that sin, but because of God's grace he covers us. *"If we confess our sins, he [God] is faithful and just and will forgive us our sins and purify us from all unrighteousness."*[99]

"If you forgive those who sin against you, your heavenly Father will forgive you. But if you refuse to forgive others, your Father will not forgive your sins."[100]

So ultimately we forgive others because we are commanded to do so and because our forgiveness depends on it! Forgiveness therefore is not an emotional response to a set of requirements that others must satisfy in acknowledging their wrongdoing. Forgiveness is a one-sided equation. We choose to forgive whether or not someone acknowledges he has hurt us. Why? Because God tells us to do so and because He knows that an unforgiving spirit stores up anger, resentment, and hatred and ultimately destroys us on all levels. Forgiving others ultimately frees us from these chains that can make us miserable. Forgiveness does not mean that we are setting others free from the consequences of their sin and need of repentance. In fact, the Bible says that when we repay our enemies with acts of kindness, it's like heaping hot coals on their head.

Should this be our goal? No! Our goal should be to love all

---

[99] 1 John 1:9
[100] Matthew 6:14

people and to be at peace with them if possible. We should pray for those who are harboring anger, resentment, and hatred that they may be set free as well.

Is there anyone you need to forgive? Anyone who stirs gut emotions when you see them or talk to them? I remember this all too well with my dad. For years I was angry with him and would experience tension in my solar plexus every time I spoke to him.

If there's someone like that in your life, pray that God will give you His power to forgive them.

If you try to do it in your own strength or, worse yet, ignore these feelings altogether, you will probably find yourself repeating this lesson often and experience the health repercussions.

3. The Principle of Earnest Prayer
Ask for God's intervention and help

Prayer is our communication with God, an essential part of our relationship with Him. Matthew Henry, who wrote in the 1600s, called prayer a letter sent from earth to heaven, just as His Word is like a love letter written to us. The power is in the One who answers prayer, who watches over us and has mercy on us. God is able to do *"immeasurably more than all we ask or imagine."*[101] If you are ill, pray for healing and pray for miracles. This is the same God who made you, who designed the human body, and who has provided miraculous recoveries throughout history.

In the book of Hosea, God describes people who have turned away from Him toward evil, and says, *"They do not cry out to me from their hearts but wail upon their beds."*[102] This is what God wants: that we would cry out to Him from our hearts about everything. If we have a relationship with Him through Jesus Christ, we can enter His presence confidently; He is our perfect, loving Father. As His Word says, He loves you with an everlasting love. He longs for communication from you. He wants us to

---

[101] Ephesians 3:20
[102] Hosea 7:14

approach Him honestly, humbly, and in our own simple words. It is as if you have a hotline to God. The Creator and Ruler of the Universe is calling and is prepared to give you His undivided attention. Are you picking up the phone to answer, or putting Him on hold while you tend to other people and activities? Nevertheless, He doesn't want us to come to Him because of duty, a program, or a list of things to do. He wants us to come to Him because we love Him.

Prayer is a mysterious process, fully understood only by God. Do we come to Him in prayer and He answers? Or does He put a desire in our hearts that moves us to pray to Him? All we know is that He has given us the responsibility to pray, and even Jesus prayed to God the Father. When we pray, what we tell Him isn't news to Him. We don't surprise Him. In fact, Jesus said that *"Your Father knows what you need before you ask Him."*[103] We can rest safely in the knowledge that we don't need to be wise enough to know what to ask for; God will pray on our behalf. *"We do not know what we ought to pray for, but the Spirit himself intercedes for us with groans that words cannot express."*[104] What an incredible thought! The Holy Spirit prays to the Father for you!

How should we pray then? Your physical position for prayer may vary according to your circumstances. People in the Bible prayed sitting, standing, kneeling, and even lying face down on the floor. Most important is coming with an attitude of reverence, the proper "position" of your mind. Prayer begins by addressing God: Lord, Father, Heavenly Father, Loving God, Lord God Almighty, even "Abba," the Aramaic word for papa. Prayer is not just an isolated time of intense interaction with God. It also is the ongoing conversation that you have with Him through the course of the day, bringing every little thing to Him. It is a way of life, rather than a required task. But it is important to set aside time each day when you are doing nothing else. It is normal to be easily distracted, caught up in the whirlwind of the day's events. Begin your session of prayer by quieting your mind—you may spend a few minutes

---

[103] Matthew 6:8
[104] Romans 8:26

129

breathing in and out slowly. Even better, spend some time in His Word first, and then reflect on it. Or you may pray as you read His Word, asking Him to open your heart and mind to grasp what He is saying to you. Some people begin their prayer session with a worshipful song or reading a psalm out loud.

What should we pray about? Everything! *"Do not be anxious about anything, but in everything, by prayer and petition, with thanksgiving, present your requests to God. And the peace of God, which transcends all understanding, will guard your hearts and your minds in Christ Jesus."*[105]

One method of prayer helps us to avoid the pattern of sessions that are merely long wish lists of what we want. Use the acrostic **ACTS** (which is the name of one of the books in the Bible): Adoration, Confession, Thanksgiving, and Supplication. Adoration is worship—praising God. Then we confess the thoughts and actions that we know aren't pleasing to Him and ask for His forgiveness. Thanksgiving in "everything" is a challenge, but becomes more possible over time as we see that even the things that seem terribly negative are actually trials that will help us grow into who He always meant us to be. Finally, supplication is the act of humbly and sincerely presenting our requests to Him. Use ACTS if it helps you to pray less selfishly. But prayer shouldn't be according to a formula, anymore than you would follow a formula when talking to a friend. Be simple, be honest, be reverent, and be real.

Remember that God will not answer your prayers based on what you deserve. He will answer based on the merit of Jesus. Jesus said, *"Until now you have not asked for anything in my name. Ask and you will receive, and your joy will be complete."*[106] When we were children and asked our parents for something, we knew we could ask because of the relationship we had with them. The relationship we have with God is based on the cross, as explained in Chapter 2. It is possible only because of Jesus. We come before God, in Christ, claiming what He did and who He is as the reason God should answer our prayers, not claiming anything about ourselves. As we

---

[105] Philippians 4:6-7
[106] John 16:24

learn more about God, we have a better idea of what can appropriately be prayed in His name. Fortunately for us, His grace will cover our mistakes and failures and lack of words. Our prayers take on a beauty of their own, even described in His Word as a fine incense floating up to Him.

Pray about anything and everything. Pray for friends, family, other believers, neighbors, and co-workers. Pray for changes in the world. Pray for help with your problems, and pray for spiritual needs. For example, you can pray that God would remove a temptation, help you to trust Him, help you to read His Word more often. You can pray that He will put love in your heart for someone you don't like. You can ask Him for the courage to tell other people about the love of Jesus Christ. You can even ask Him to help you treat your spouse better and more respectfully. God tells us to ask others to pray for us, too. If it would humble you to ask for prayer, that's all the more reason to do it! Always be faithful when you tell others that you will pray for them. We have to be careful not to say lightly, "I'll pray for you," and then forget such an awesome responsibility. Keep on praying for yourself and others, like the persistent widow in Luke 18:1-8.

God's Word contains many examples of prayer. You'll find many prayers in the book of Psalms in the Old Testament. They are honest and filled with raw emotions (both positive and negative). The people, who wrote them, under the direction of the Holy Spirit, honestly expressed many questions, thoughts, and feelings, including joy, anger, frustration, fear, and sorrow. Many believers have made it a habit to read a psalm each day.

4) The Principle of Submission
Submit every choice and decision to God's direction

Submission? Does your ego flare up at the very thought? That little surge of emotion is a sign that the ego dies a long, hard death. Deep inside we still want to be our own god. If you have a relationship with the living God, you can turn to Him for guidance in every matter, including the will power to eat well and exercise, the step of obedience to forgive others, and the best way to honor your spouse or parents in every situation. Should you make that remark? Should you remain silent? Should you stay with an existing employer, buy a new house, or seek help from a particular doctor or minister? Ask God.

Trust in the LORD with all your heart and lean not on your own understanding; in all your ways acknowledge him, and he will make your paths straight.[107]

Submit your plans, questions, and decisions to God. The first place to figure out His will for you is in the Bible. His Word is completely true and trustworthy. In contrast, our desires can distort our view of the truth. In addition to His Word, if you have a relationship with Him, His laws are written on your heart and His Holy Spirit speaks to you in a still, small voice. He speaks to you through other believers and through circumstances, as well. Submit your decisions to Him. Listen and watch for His response. Then do what He says.

Why doesn't God always answer my prayers? There are many answers to this question. The first is, we don't know. His mind is so much greater than ours, and we understand so little about life's purpose. The second is, sometimes His answer is "No." But beyond that, there are a number of reasons given in His Word. Sometimes God is putting us through a difficult experience in order to make us more spiritually mature (see James 1:2-4). Sometimes our motives may be wrong. Instead of our highest goal being to serve God, our desire may be to live a self-centered life: *"When you ask, you do not receive, because you ask with wrong motives, that you may spend what you get on your pleasures."*[108] Sometimes we may not believe that God is going to answer our prayers, and this lack of faith interferes with the answer:

But when he asks, he must believe and not doubt, because he

---

[107] Proverbs 3:5-6
[108] James 4:3

who doubts is like a wave of the sea, blown and tossed by the wind. That man should not think he will receive anything from the Lord; he is a double-minded man, unstable in all he does.[109]

Remember, though, that even if we can't expect God to answer a faithless prayer, He is a merciful God who can choose to overlook our lack of trust and our doubts.

We may not receive an answer to prayer because we are consciously holding on to a sin in our hearts (see Psalm 66:18). For this reason, it's wise to begin a session of prayer with an invitation to God to examine our hearts:

Search me, O God, and know my heart; test me and know my anxious thoughts. See if there is any offensive way in me, and lead me in the way everlasting.[110]

Our attitudes toward people and our behavior toward them can reveal a state of mind that is not conducive to honest prayer or to the answer we want. For example, husbands are instructed to be considerate as they live with their wives, *"so that nothing will hinder your prayers."*[111]

Finally, God may not answer a prayer in the way we want simply because our request, no matter how good it may seem, does not go along with His will:

This is the confidence we have in approaching God: that if we ask anything according to his will, he hears us. And if we know that he hears us—whatever we ask—we know that we have what we asked of him.[112]

After all, if God knows that you are asking for something that would be dangerous for you, or that isn't part of His plan, or that

---

[109] James 1:6-7
[110] Psalm 139:23-24
[111] 1 Peter 3:7
[112] 1John 5:14-15

isn't supposed to happen for another few years, or that would keep you from becoming the person that He is growing you to be, or that wouldn't fit into a wonderful plan He has for someone else—would you want Him to give you what you want or to override your request? He may not always answer your prayer in the way that you would like. He will always answer it in the way that is best for you. I can recount several times when God has said no or closed a door that I thought was opening, and now I look back and see how limited my vision was or how God always knows what is best! I am learning to just pray, "Lord, Your will be done in every situation."

5. The Principle of Gratitude
Receive God's blessings with thanksgiving

We come to God with nothing to offer Him. He fills our empty hands with showers of blessings. The universe is so large and we are so small. It is a wonder that the Creator even cares about us, as David wrote thousands of years ago:

When I consider your heavens, the work of your fingers, the moon and the stars, which you have set in place, what is man that you are mindful of him?[113]

Yet, He gives us Himself. He gave us His Son and His Word. If we accept Him, He gives us eternal life. He gives us our every talent, every skill, every penny, and every friend and loved one. The rain falling on our upturned faces, the rainbow that breaks through the clouds, the starry night skies are all gifts to us.

One of God's amazing traits is His creativity, as demonstrated in the great range of colors, flowers, herbs, leaves, fish, birds, and the great variety of delicious foods He has provided. He could have furnished the entire world with one plain, gray utilitarian fruit to supply the required vitamins in our diet. Instead, He lavished on us

---

[113] Psalm 8:3-4

luscious, sweet melons, plump purple berries, fuzzy peaches, and hundreds of other delicious plants for our health and enjoyment. Life isn't meant to be an experience of deprivation. God has provided everything we need for a rich, full, enjoyable life, regardless of our specific circumstances. Remember this as you design your health program and even more so as you "design" your life. You may need to eliminate some things that you used to enjoy, but the rewards will be great. Enjoy what you do have and be grateful. Each day, reflect on the things for which you are thankful. Some people make a list in a daily journal. Even better is to come before God every day to thank Him.

6. The Principle of a Surrendered Life
Live God's way instead of your own

Therefore, I urge you, brothers, in view of God's mercy, to offer your bodies as living sacrifices, holy and pleasing to God— this is your spiritual act of worship. Do not conform any longer to the pattern of this world, but be transformed by the renewing of your mind. Then you will be able to test and approve what God's will is—his good, pleasing and perfect will. [114]

God's Word is clear: You'll never know God's perfect will for you until you're willing to surrender: to give your life to Him, to stop living for yourself, your ego, and to start living His way. Ask yourself this: If God created you, if He created the universe, if He established reality, what point is there to living any other way? It would be foolish, wouldn't it? God tells us that having an authentic relationship with Him is not just a matter of having some rosy feelings. Jesus is blunt on this subject: ***"If you love me, you will obey what I command."*** [115]

This quote from God's Word begins with the word "Therefore." Why? Because all the preceding chapters in the

---

[114] Romans 12:1-2
[115] John 14:15

apostle Paul's letter to the Romans spelled out what God has done for us, how He has done it all for us, and paid the price necessary for us to have eternal life. In light of what He has done, what should my response be? To give my life to Him. He paid for it; it should be His now.

What will He do with your life if you give it to Him? He will do what is best for you. He has only your best interests in mind when He tells you to live life according to His instructions, which are found in His Book. He asks you to follow Him, to trust Him, and to leave the consequences to Him. When you live God's way, much of the stress, tension, anxiety, and confusion immediately vanishes. You can experience authentic peace. Jesus said:

"Come to me, all you who are weary and burdened, and I will give you rest. Take my yoke upon you and learn from me, for I am gentle and humble in heart, and you will find rest for your souls. For my yoke is easy and my burden is light."[116]

A yoke was a bar of wood used to join two oxen together, so that they could pull a load. Often a young ox would be yoked to an older, larger one. If the younger one struggled to go his own way, each step was difficult and in the wrong direction. The more he learned to walk in step with the older ox, the easier, less painful, and more productive his journey would be.

Jesus calls us to take His yoke upon us, to learn from Him, to walk in step with Him, to unburden ourselves of the load we've been carrying of ego, wrongdoing, sin, anxiety, fear, resentment, stress, and envy. Instead, we should carry only His burden, doing His will. In contrast to our own heavy burden, His burden is light—to obey Someone who loves you. Notice that He doesn't offer His yoke, His light burden, or His "rest" to just anyone. His offer is to those who are weary and burdened—in other words, those who have acknowledged their self-afflicted encumbrance. Only when you admit to carrying this burden can you be free of it. This is the person who has awakened to the truths of Chapter 2.

---

[116] Matthew 11:28-30

When you become, in effect, yoked to Jesus, He works with you, leading you step by step. He is patient and will take whatever time is necessary to grow you spiritually. The result is "rest for your soul."

Let's review just three areas of life and see what might be involved in surrendering these to God. As we do, consider the implications for the stress in your life, and ultimately your health.

Make God your top priority. In the first of the Ten Commandments, God said, *"You shall have no other gods before me."*[117] And in the second commandment, God tells us not to worship idols. When our modern mind sees the words "other gods" and "idols," we picture superstitious people worshiping a stone carving or something equally powerless. We deceive ourselves. Anything that we put before God in our hearts, our energies, or our decision-making is our idol, our other god. God sees this behavior as a rejection and betrayal of Him. Do you have another god? How about money (examine your checkbook for your priorities), the stock market, Sunday football games, what people think of you, sexual relationships, your career, your intellect, or even yourself? What comes first on your list of things to do? What keeps you from surrendering to God? Your priorities in life will become clearer; they will no longer be a source of confusion and anxiety if they are firmly established on the foundation of what God wants. In every decision, defer to Him.

Be truthful. Have an open, confessing heart. Live a transparent life. Before having a personal relationship with God, you must admit to yourself and to Him just what your true nature is. Now that you've done that, make it a practice to regularly confess your wrongdoings and faults to Him, and in many cases to another believer, too. Obviously, you shouldn't tell people the gory details about things you have done wrong, or share information that would make them uncomfortable, but never use this as an excuse for covering up your own wrongdoing. Stop hiding your addictions. Be honest when you file your taxes. Give up deception; don't mislead people or even just allow them to make false assumptions. Reject

---

[117] Exodus 20:3

the white lies that so many people depend on to function in their jobs and relationships. God is offended by lies of any type. One bonus: If you no longer tell white lies, you won't have the stress of keeping all of your facts straight! Be accountable to others. If you feel compelled to hide parts of your life from people and don't let them know where you are, whom you are with, or what you are doing, something is wrong. Would you feel comfortable if all the people in your life met in one room and compared notes? You should! Examine your heart in the presence of God. Turn from your wrongdoings and experience forgiveness and true freedom.

Control your tongue. God tells us to *"be quick to listen, slow to speak and slow to become angry."*[118] Think of the reduction of stress in your life if you never were to speak unkind words, if you never were to talk about people behind their backs, if you never were to speak hastily, boastfully, or in anger. Some of us have the same problem, but in a different direction. We say "Yes" when we should say "No." We compromise the truth so that people will like us. We go beyond the requirements of kindness and compromise our principles by approving of things that we know are wrong. We quickly agree to projects, relationships, commitments, and decisions without consulting God first, and deeply regret it later. With this, as with everything else, we need so much help from God! There is virtually nothing in our lives as hard to control as the tongue. But imagine the peace you'll have when you don't need to repair the damage your words have caused yourself and others.

The Principle of a Surrendered Life is especially important to people with addictions—to food, shopping, power, money, sex, drugs, alcohol, television, or even to being busy. When you persist in doing things that damage your life and can't stop, you may have an addiction. The damage may come in the form of heart disease or ruined relationships or even just wasted time that leads to a wasted life. Addictions never satisfy. If you are addicted to food, there will never be enough. If you are addicted to alcohol, you will never find that drink that makes you say, "At last I've found it and I'll never need another." An addiction to money won't end with someone

---

[118] James 1:19

saying, "Now I have enough." God's Word describes this as having *"a continual lust for more."*[119]

We need to learn to take our feelings and problems to God, instead of to our addictions. Rather than burying ourselves in the addiction, we throw ourselves headlong into the love of God. The surrendered life may be a frightening prospect for those of us who are under the control of these addictions. Part of the reason is that we know our addictions have left behind so many piles of wreckage. To turn away from addiction and toward God would mean to come out of denial and deal with the consequences of our addictions, something we want to avoid at literally any cost. We would also need to learn to handle life God's way, and that requires relinquishing control. It's like standing on a dock, afraid to dive into the water. If only we knew how warm, soothing, and pleasurable that water is! We may be accustomed to reacting to events and people around us with anger, resentment, and fear. Instead of acknowledging that these reactions have their source in a self-centered part of our hearts, we blame the people around us and then medicate ourselves with our addiction. It's a vicious cycle—we set ourselves up in situations and relationships that are certain to provide us with the excuses we need to medicate ourselves again. How complicated! How exhausting! The effects on our health can be devastating. But, when we "let go and let God," His grace will stun us with its incredible power to heal, to help, and to satisfy.

7. The Principle of Meekness
Soften your heart and quietly yield to God

Meekness helps us to react to God, to people, and to our circumstances in a radically new and clearly less stressful way. Meekness is a gift of the Holy Spirit, meaning that it is a characteristic that the Holy Spirit develops in us as we immerse our lives in God and follow His example. An old-fashioned word sometimes translated "gentleness," meekness is related to humility,

---

[119] Ephesians 4:19

but it has a deeper meaning.

A meek person's heart has been softened, and his will has been tamed by God. As Matthew Henry wrote hundreds of years ago in his book *The Quest for a Meek and Quiet Spirit,* the Romans called a meek man "manu assuetus," which means "used to the hand." This reference to the taming of a wild horse is a picture of the man who walks with God: accustomed to the hand of God, yielding to His will, following His guidance, and desiring to walk in step with Him. He doesn't startle at God's touch, resist, or rebel; instead, he quietly and agreeably follows His lead. Matthew Henry describes meekness toward God as "the easy and quiet submission of the soul to God's whole will, however He makes it known." Meekness makes us soft and workable so that God's Word can have an effect on us. Henry has beautiful metaphors for meekness: If we are meek, we are like a sheet of fresh, white paper ready for God to write anything He wants on us. We are like soft wax, ready to receive the impression of His seal.

A meek person has been humbled by his awareness of what God has done for him. A meek person has grasped how holy and pure God is, how powerful, just, wise, and all knowing. The Bible says, *"Our God is a consuming fire."*[120] When we stand before this truly awesome God someday, we will not refer to Him as "the man upstairs," or chatter on about how good we think we've been and that our wrongdoings were really someone else's fault. We will see His majesty and glory, and our mouths will be shut. We will fall on our faces before Him. We will be filled with reverence and awe. Meek men and women carry this reverence and awe in their hearts as they walk through each day.

Meekness is, first and foremost, meekness toward God. But the truly meek person will also display meekness toward other people. Jesus is the perfect example of meekness. *"When they hurled their insults at him, he did not retaliate; when he suffered, he made no threats. Instead, he entrusted himself to him who judges*

---

[120] Hebrews 12:29

justly. "[121] His goal wasn't to defend himself, to impress others, or to insist on His rights. His goal was to please His Father. He wasn't passive or afraid of confrontation, but He saw the big picture. He could look at people and see that they were slaves to their own fear, selfishness, and wrongdoing, and that they needed to know God. They needed someone to save them. We should pray for the ability to see people through God's eyes and pray, too, for help in following Jesus' example in seeking only to please the Father. When we are sure of our purpose in life and fix our eyes on His example, we will find that people and events cannot provoke us to anger and other emotions quite so easily.

Let us fix our eyes on Jesus, the author and perfecter of our faith, who for the joy set before him endured the cross, scorning its shame, and sat down at the right hand of the throne of God. Consider him who endured such opposition from sinful men, so that you will not grow weary and lose heart.[122]

When we are meek, we can see all events as being under God's control. This too can give us an entirely different perspective on life. We learn to give up arguing with God, complaining about His will, and telling Him what to do. As we begin to have an inkling of how powerful, holy, and just He is, we realize how foolish, insane, and wrong it is to fight Him for control of our lives. We turn over the reins to Him, or, to use a more modern analogy, we give up the driver's seat to Him. He knows what is best for us, He wants what is best for us, and He even knows the best timing for each event in our lives. We see that difficult times, difficult people, and even suffering cannot come into our lives without His allowing it. He doesn't cause evil, as we discussed in Chapter 2. But where evil exists, He is able to use it for good.

For example, someone may speak harshly to you. It was wrong for that person to treat you that way, but if you are meek, you will see that God may be allowing you to have that experience because

---

[121] 1 Peter 2:23
[122] Hebrews 12:2-3

He wants you to be more patient, loving, or humble. He may also be showing you how people have felt when you have spoken harshly to them. He uses the experiences of our lives, both positive and negative, to shape us, to chisel away at the parts of us that aren't like Him. To use an analogy from God's Word, God brings people and experiences into our lives to prune us, as a vine is carefully pruned. The pruning may be painful at the time, but the result is growth, health, and a fruitful life.

As the Holy Spirit develops meekness in us, we begin to realize that we don't have the right to create an agenda for life or for other people. We don't view each experience or relationship as an opportunity to meet our own needs. Instead, we see it as an opportunity to serve the living God. This attitude develops over a lifetime of knowing Him. Without meekness, think of the emotions— the anger, resentment, frustration, disappointment, worry, and fear— that flood us when circumstances are not going our way or as we had hoped, when the behavior of others doesn't meet our expectations. But, if we are following God's agenda each day instead of our own, if we are "used to the hand" and following His lead, that enormous burden of our own agenda can be lifted from us. What relief and peace that brings to our mind, body, and spirit!

How do meekness and anger connect with health? The ability to control anger and express the reasons for it properly have been associated with lower levels of bad cholesterol and higher levels of good cholesterol. Also, anger floods the body with stress hormones. An attitude of anger assaults our cells and organs, especially the liver, on a continuous basis, contributing to hypertension, muscle tension, a weakened immune system, and digestive problems. As we grow in the Lord and He develops this quality of meekness within us, the assault can finally diminish, and even cease.

8. The Principle of Contentment
Be truly content with what a faithful and sovereign God has given us

Much of the stress in our lives is caused, directly or indirectly, by lack of contentment. You should not be content with the dysfunctions in your life, but as you strive to improve things, you must begin to enjoy the journey. Otherwise you will always be miserable! The Principle of Contentment provides us with inner calm and appreciation for the great blessings we have already received. Keenly aware that we come to God with nothing to offer, we joyfully appreciate the blessings, the mercy and grace He has showered upon us. We can savor each moment of life. We can say, "What You have given me, Lord, is enough," and not be distracted by the sense of emptiness, want, greed, ambition, and even loneliness that plagues so many. In the stages of ego, contentment is impossible. We chase after temporary things that provide no satisfaction. We are oppressed by our own covetousness, the feeling that what we have, or are, isn't enough, and that we deserve what someone else has. Lack of contentment causes a kind of stress that slowly eats away at us. In the awakened state, we trust God to provide what He knows we need. Trusting God allows us to escape the physical effects of anxiety.

Contentment's sister is acceptance. We can be content, and accept the people and events around us, when we fully realize how thoroughly God is in control. Nothing happens that wasn't created or allowed by God. If you have entered into a relationship with the living God, He chose you before the creation of the world to live for Him and to be in a loving relationship with Him. Keenly aware of your faults and weaknesses, your selfish motivations, your fears and genetic predispositions, He set out a path before you. He will bring into your life exactly what is needed to draw you close to Him and make you more like Him. When you turn away from Him, forget Him, or walk out of step with Him, He will do what is necessary to pull you back. He will find you, wherever you go. Nothing that happens to you takes Him by surprise. The safest place on earth is in the center of God's will. Resting on this knowledge, we can look at our circumstances, from the smallest irritation to the most frightening catastrophe, and know we are held in His loving hands.

However, we are not puppets; God allows us to use our free will. The interplay between God's control and our free will is beyond our ability to understand. At the same time that we trust Him to be in charge and to help us, we must accept complete responsibility for all of our actions and their consequences. An unwed, pregnant teenager, who was receiving misguided spiritual advice from an older woman, said with a sigh, "Yes, I see now that this pregnancy happened for a reason." That's true! It happened for the reason that she chose a completely wrong path in life and made a series of decisions that were destructive to herself, the baby, and her family. By clinging to vague, pseudo-spiritual statements, she was attempting to find comfort and absolve herself of responsibility for what she had done.

This is the egotistic approach to life. It enables us to continue down self-deceptive, destructive paths. Confessing the truth and accepting 100 percent of the responsibility for our actions is the only thing that will set us free and move us into spiritual maturity. The sinful thoughts and actions of humanity constantly bring more pain and suffering into this world, setting into motion millions of negative chains of events. We shouldn't throw up our hands and merely say, "Oh well, I guess this is all God's will." He is not responsible for evil and suffering. But even our wrongdoings and wrong choices can't be made unless He allows them. He will use them to accomplish His will, although the consequences of our choices will be painful. Once you have a relationship with God, you can choose to avoid a great deal of pain by simply obeying Him, rather than choosing the most painful, long, and torturous path through each experience in life. The path of peace is found only by walking in His light, obeying Him.

Contentment, discontentment, and complacency are three different states of mind. The contented person is God-centered; he tries to have God's perspective and priorities, taking action in obedience to God and His Word. We change what we can, if we should. Otherwise, we accept what we have or wait for God's timing before making changes. The discontented person, who is in the stages of ego, focuses energies on complaining and wanting. He changes little or nothing; if he does make changes, it is without God's direction. These feelings and activities will never bring contentment, only continued restlessness and a critical spirit. The complacent person, who is also in the stages of ego, does not seek God's wisdom or direction but settles for whatever is there.

For example, a young woman is employed by a company that treats its workers badly. The contented person will see that it is possible to do something about it: quit the job. She will pray and ask God if she should quit. If she believes that He wants her to quit, she will move ahead to do that, in His timing. If she believes that He wants her to stay, she won't quit, but she also won't complain. She will see that God wants her there and she will have a sense of peace as she carries out His will for her. The discontented person may stay at the job and complain incessantly to her co-workers. Or she may leave the job without praying first, and regardless of where she works next, she will not have peace. She will most likely see her condition as someone else's fault, no matter what situation she is in. The complacent person will remain in the job, not because God has told her to, but perhaps because she is too lazy or fearful to make the change. Only one of these three people will have peace.

One indication that discontent doesn't come from truly needing something is that discontent runs rampant throughout the United States, where most of us have much more than the rest of the world. Advertising is geared to push our buttons, to make us feel needy, incomplete, and dissatisfied. Shopping centers and store aisles have eye-catching displays of products that end up in a garage sale a year or two later. We actually begin to believe that we'd be happier if we owned a different car. The goal is to make us feel that life would be better if only we had that product or experience, but these things never really satisfy, do they? Our aim should be to be like the apostle Paul, who wrote, *"I have learned to be content whatever the circumstances."*[123] Paul knew what the apostle John knew, that *"The world and its desires pass away, but the man who does the will of God lives forever."*[124]

How much more will you need to feel content? How many more toys do your children need? Are you teaching them

---

[123] Philippians 4:11
[124] 1 John 2:17

145

contentment and the joys of simple, useful possessions, of nature, and of library storybooks? What do you allow into your life that only serves to make you discontent: catalogs, television, decorating magazines, the real estate section of the newspaper, window shopping, restaurant reviews, shopping on the Internet? How many projects have you taken on, how many books that you'd hoped would change your life? If you feel more content and satisfied with your life when you've finished, by all means, continue to use these things. It's not that these things are bad in and of themselves, but maybe they preoccupy too much of your time. On the other hand, if you're left with a discontented feeling, maybe it's time to cut them out. You won't miss them; your life will be full without them. In fact, you will find you have more time for your family, more time for inspirational music, more time for new hobbies, more time for exercise, and most importantly more time to spend with God and to learn His ways.

Contentment applies to much more than possessions, money, and time. Are you content with your weight if you are healthy? Are you content with your face, age, race, curly or straight hair, or gender? Are you content with being single? Are you content with your husband or wife, or is your spouse well aware of the fact that you are dissatisfied with him or her in many ways? What percentage of your conversation each day is devoted to complaining about other people, your family, your job, your house, yourself? As stated earlier, there are times to seek change in your life, but we know, deep in our hearts, that God wants us to learn to be content with, and even thankful for, everything in our lives except sin.

This becomes easier and clearer as we allow Him to be Lord of our lives. In the final analysis, it is a relationship with the living God that brings contentment. All else falls short. Every attempt on our own to find serenity, simplicity, or peace will ultimately fail. Only God Himself and knowing Him fill our hearts to overflowing. As you turn your resources (time, energy, money, talents, possessions) toward God's priorities, you will not only find contentment, but also discover the exhilaration and delight that come from walking in step with God and accomplishing your life's mission. Ask for His help to redirect your life toward one of contentment. He will provide everything you need to do what He created you for. *"And God is able to make all grace abound to you, so that in all things at all times, having all that you need, you will abound in every good work."*[125]

9. The Principle of a Quiet Life
Have a quiet heart and a quiet life

God's Word tells us, *"Make it your ambition to lead a quiet life, to mind your own business and to work with your hands."*[126] Not a boring life but a quiet one!

God would like to redirect your efforts toward quietness. With all the noise that the world makes, clamoring for our attention, it will indeed require ambition, devotion, and focus to create a quiet life. All too often, we can agree with the suffering Job of the Bible, who said, *"I have no peace, no quietness; I have no rest, but only turmoil."*[127] In contrast, the person with a quiet life can have serenity, a calm heart, and an undistracted, peaceful mind. A quiet life is only possible for the person who has quietness on the inside as well as the outside. An angry man locked alone in a padded cell may be surrounded by silence, but he will not have a quiet heart or a quiet life. What disturbs our quiet? Envy, greed, competition, gossip, resentment, anger, fear, anxiety, and not trusting God. These things come from within us and from how we have chosen to react to our circumstances and to people. They are a major contributing factor to the release of stress hormones. God can liberate us from all of these reactions if we let Him.

Quietness is different from emptiness. The quiet life may be full of music, laughter, nature, worship, adventure, and friendship. The Bible says that a life immersed in the pursuit of God and following His ways is a life filled with joy and freedom. *"For the*

---

[125] 2 Corinthians 9:8
[126] 1 Thessalonians 4:11
[127] Job 3:26

poor, every day brings trouble; for the happy heart, life is a continual feast."[128] "Poor" is not referring to financial deprivation, but to the soul deprived of refreshment by God and His Spirit.

As you get to know God better, you'll discover He has a great sense of humor; He doesn't require a dour personality to follow Him. The Spirit-filled life described in Chapter 2 is the only way of truly fulfilling and enjoying the life that God has given us. If you find yourself being legalistic about your faith—always serious, seldom cheerful—I would suggest that you hang out with children for a while. Perhaps volunteering in a children's ministry will help you to recognize the child-like faith that God calls us to and start to laugh a little more. Don't get me wrong, the message of the gospel is serious, the consequences of sin deadly. Nonetheless, many believers are too serious, their lives missing happiness and joy.

Knowing God, trusting and obeying Him will give us a quiet heart, as described in the other 11 principles, and a life overflowing with joy! The Principle of a Quiet Life helps us to turn from the world's attempts to capture our minds and lives, and to devote ourselves to hearing God's voice and enjoying the life He has given us, as we perform the work He has provided.

A quiet life most often requires us to mind our own business. Jesus knew what His business was. He said and did only what His Father told Him to do. Ultimately, that is our business, too. Look not to what other people think, act, and say, but to what God says, and to what He wants you to do today. Avoid the emotional roller coaster that many people around you are on. Share God's love with them, but be careful not to get trapped listening to endless complaints or participating in gossip. Has it really ever helped you or the other person? In each situation, pray that God will show you the difference between sacrificial love, which He requires of you, and enabling, which merely helps people to stay in their current self-destructive state. Minding your own business does not mean to keep silent about the liberating truth found in God's Word. The Bible says, *"All Scripture is inspired by God and is useful to teach us what is true and to make us realize what is wrong in our*

---

[128] Proverbs 15:15 New Living Translation

lives. It straightens us out and teaches us to do what is right. "[129]
If you are called to correct someone, be careful to do it in love, humility, and the power of the Holy Spirit. Always confront the person directly to try to resolve any issue before enlisting the help of others. The Bible gives clear instruction on how to handle every situation you may face.

Minding your own business may also mean simplifying your life. What adds to the tranquility in your life? What adds to the turmoil? If you have joined a church, you may even find that many activities and ministries separate your family and add to the busyness of life instead of leading you to God. Take a fresh look at your entire schedule and bring it all before God. A man who has devoted himself to the procurement of wealth may have a life that is busy, intense, and fast; none of these qualities have any value in themselves. In fact, his devotion to money may come at the cost of family, friendships, health, and serenity. But a man with a quiet life may have a happy, united family and a life that is rich with simple pleasures. *"Better a dry crust with peace and quiet than a house full of feasting, with strife."*[130]

If you have a relationship with the living God, His Holy Spirit lives within you, and a quiet life will help you hear His voice. God's voice is sometimes unmistakable, startling, and undeniable. Our circumstances may shout His intentions at us. But usually, His voice is quiet and gentle. He often speaks to us as we read His Word, opening our eyes to things we never noticed before, opening our hearts to new understandings. *"Be still, and know that I am God,"* says the Lord.[131]

10. The Principle of Fellowship
Develop emotional intimacy with God and those who love Him

A number of studies and physicians have made us aware of the

---

[129] 2 Timothy 3:16
[130] Proverbs 17:1
[131] Psalm 46:10

connection between close relationships, particularly in a group setting, and health. They clearly demonstrate a dramatically positive effect on health when people meet at least weekly with others who are going through similar experiences, and share a form of emotional intimacy with them.

For example, Dr. David Spiegel at Stanford University School of Medicine studied two groups of women with metastatic breast cancer. One received standard medical care for their condition; the other group also took part in a weekly 90-minute support group. Five years later, the women who participated in the weekly support group had twice the survival rate of the other group. At Yale University, patients who were about to receive an angiography (which viewed their coronary arteries) were questioned about their relationships. The more loved and supported those patients felt, the lower the degree of atherosclerosis (clogged arteries). Risk factors such as age, sex, high blood pressure, smoking, genetics, and high cholesterol were taken into consideration, and the results were true even independently of these risk factors. The most successful program for alcoholism is Alcoholics Anonymous, the cornerstone of which is frequent meetings with fellow alcoholics, where participants speak openly and honestly.

We can go even deeper when we have a relationship with the living God. The Principle of Fellowship offers us emotional intimacy with people who love God and with God Himself. Fellowship for the believer is a close relationship with other believers who share your life's purpose, your reason for being. Fellowship is based on a common knowledge and experience of God, and exhibited in honesty, confession, accountability, prayer, teaching, communion, sharing, and love in action. It is not only essential to the experience of someone who has a relationship with God, but also *evidence* of it. God's Word tells us to love one another, sincerely, deeply, from the heart and as He loves us. *"Be imitators of God, therefore, as dearly loved children and live a life of love, just as Christ loved us and gave himself up for us."*[132]

Obviously, when God speaks of love, He isn't merely

---

[132] Ephesians 5:1-2

describing a feeling. In the awakened state, we submit ourselves to God's definition of love, His requirements for a loving relationship, and we depend on Him for the strength to do it. A loving relationship calls for forgiveness when we don't want to forgive, apologizing when we are certain the other person is just as wrong as we are, confessing faults we'd rather keep hidden, sharing when we don't have enough, and being accountable to others for how we live when we'd rather it was no one else's business. It calls for loving the unlovely: people who are irritating, shockingly different in their personal tastes, socially unacceptable (but accepted by God), politically incorrect, and not quite up to our standards. They, like you, are constantly moving in and out of the ego and awakened stages in various areas of their lives. The rewards of this kind of fellowship are spectacular: spiritual growth; the profoundly spiritual experience of worshiping and praising God together; the exhilaration of knowing God together and talking about Him; having others share with you, take care of you, pray with you, and encourage you. When you aren't growing spiritually, someone will inspire you with his or her example. When you are brokenhearted, failing, or suffering, a brother or sister will lift you up. You'll also have the experience of laughter, joy, and feasting together. God's Word says, *"A merry heart does good, like medicine."*[133]

Something mystical happens when we become believers that unites us to other believers. We will not know its full meaning until we are in heaven. There is no suggestion that we will be absorbed into one another or into God. On the contrary, we each have, and will have, our own individual, loving relationship with God, and we will each have our own spiritual body. But when we become believers we can no longer be on our own, with some sort of special, individualistic, self-made religion of one. We become part of something.

God's Word uses metaphors to give our limited minds a picture of our relationship to other believers. We are described as being part of a "body," the body of Christ. We can't function as believers

---

[133] Proverbs 17:22 New King James Version

unless we are part of this body any more than a hand that is amputated can still clap. We are also described as the "bride of Christ," being prepared so that we will be a beautiful bride, ready for an absolutely incredible celebration of a wedding when we are reunited with Him. We are also described as a "nation," and it is true that, along with other believers, we are not really living in our homeland. Our homeland is heaven and the soon to be renewed earth. Until God's will be fully done on earth as it is in heaven, we need to obey the laws of this country and more importantly God's will.

We are described as sheep who are part of a flock. Jesus is our Shepherd. We are part of an "assembly," and are commanded not to forsake our regular meeting together. Before we became believers, there was nothing that tied us together, but God says that now we are "the people of God." We are even described as *living stones* who *are being built into a spiritual house.* [134] "Church" isn't a building. We are the church. Our thoughts may be caught up in looking at how different we think we are from other believers. Our egos will rebel against the idea that we absolutely must become part of the body of believers by attending a church. But, in the awakened state, we move past that to an understanding that part of surrendering to God is to obey Him in this matter, too, and to make the sacrifices necessary to learn to really love our brothers and sisters.

God has a plan for His people that is beyond our limited imaginations, and it begins with finding other people who have a relationship with Him and who believe His Word exactly as it is written, who want to walk with Him, His way. Like Him, we must look past the surface and see that these other believers, no matter how different they may seem, are simply forgiven sinners like us. His Word is full of "one another" phrases that tell us how to treat other believers. *"Be completely humble and gentle; be patient, bearing with one another in love."* [135] *"Love one another deeply,*

---

[134] 1 Peter 2:5
[135] Ephesians 4:2

from the heart."[136] The assumption made throughout God's Word is that every believer will live his life and walk his walk in close fellowship with other believers. For sure we'll have differences in the way we interpret some scriptures, but as my current pastor professes and I agree with—unity in the essentials, diversity in the non-essentials. The essentials are crystal clear: We are all sinners needing the saving grace of Jesus Christ, the Son of God who became flesh, lived a sinless life, died on the cross for our sins, and was resurrected to sit at the right hand of His Father in heaven. Any one who believes this and receives Him will be saved.

Further rewarding is the knowledge that God has said, *"The Lord is near to all who call on him, to all who call on him in truth."*[137] Fellowship with God is without parallel in the human experience. When we draw close to Him, we are able to tap into a life-changing joy that flows from an ongoing relationship with the living God. He comforts us in our sorrows, encourages us in our difficulties, and leads us into amazing relationships and adventures. He meets with us in a quiet place inside us, when our hearts are laid wide open before Him and He, the Creator of the universe, tenderly ministers to us. When asked what the greatest commandment was, Jesus replied, *"Love the Lord your God with all your heart and with all your soul and with all your mind."*[138] How do we draw close to Him? How do we learn to love Him? Through prayer, meditating on His Word, learning about Him from other believers, obeying Him, praising Him, worshiping Him, confessing our wrongdoings to Him and receiving His forgiveness, and walking through each day with Him. Obedience, a word the ego hates, cannot be ignored. When we walk in darkness, rather than walking His way, we cut ourselves off from fellowship with Him. We can't pretend to love Him if we don't care to do what He tells us. Thank God for His mercy, His help, and His forgiveness!

As we get to know Him, we begin to see people and events more and more through His eyes. As we read His Word, in a meek

---

[136] 1 Peter 1:22
[137] Psalm 145:18
[138] Matthew 22:37

and openhearted way, He changes us. We begin to see what it really means to love others, and we begin to learn how it feels to be truly loved.

11. The Principle of Compassionate Service
Humbly serve others just as Jesus gave Himself for you

One evening many years ago in Jerusalem a man who had the power to calm storms at sea and to raise the dead back to life knelt before a group of sinful men. He knew their hearts; He knew that within hours these men whom He called His friends would desert Him when He needed them the most. Nevertheless, He poured water into a basin and with His own hands washed their filthy feet, drying them with the towel that was wrapped around His waist. He said, *"Now that I, your Lord and Teacher, have washed your feet, you also should wash one another's feet."*[139]

Jesus' example then and soon after, at the cross, taught us to serve one another, even if the task is lowly, dirty, and menial, even if the task requires sacrifice of our time, our money, or our own needs. Do we do this because the person deserves it? No, we do it with the same type of love that caused God to help us when we didn't deserve it. Tenderly serving other believers and our neighbors is not only an integral part of our relationship with God, but also essential to good health. The Principle of Compassionate Service brings us out of ourselves. It pulls our focus away from stress and frustration, and brings us the great blessing of performing the good works that God created us to do. Self-esteem is a false and shallow goal, tied to the ego. In the awakened state, we can have something so much better: the awareness on a deep, inner level that we are loved by God and have a significant, unique purpose in life. Even if we are paralyzed or bedridden with chronic pain or illness, we can serve others in the most meaningful, important ways: praying for them, encouraging them, or even ministering to them on Internet message boards. No one else on

---

[139] John 13:14

earth can achieve what God has created you to do.

Bringing our physical health under the direction of God will not completely prevent disease and suffering. Some of the wisest, most generous, and humble people who have a close relationship with God endure great physical suffering every day of their lives. This is a hard path for anyone. But God tells us that He works everything for the good in the lives of those who love Him. Your suffering may have the higher purpose of teaching something to the people around you, such as leading your loved ones to a greater dependency on God.

Learning to offer up our suffering to God is a lesson that virtually everyone finds difficult. Even in those cases where suffering is clearly the result of poor choices, the anguish is just as deep. We, too, make poor choices in many areas of our lives. Our wrong steps may not be in the area of health; they may involve relationships, money, or career, and it is only God's mercy that keeps us from the consequences. We must remember this, and when we meet people who are suffering we should offer compassion and service rather than judgment.

"Compassion" means "suffering with." You share their suffering and don't feel superior to them. Some best-selling authors today suggest that if someone is sick, he or she has desired it on some level. Beware of using this philosophy to judge others. This is just a new, psychological twist on the so-called "friends" that Job encountered who told him that his suffering was caused by his secret sins. Their words angered God, who made it clear in His Word that they were wrong. Jesus encountered a man who had been blind since birth. His followers asked Him, *"Who sinned, this man or his parents, that he was born blind?"* Jesus replied that it wasn't the man's sins or his parents' sins that caused the blindness. *"This happened so that the work of God might be displayed in his life."*[140] He then reached forward and healed the man.

What a beautiful purpose for your life, too, that God might display His work in you.

---

[140] John 9:2-3

12. The Principle of Eternal Priority
Put God's Great Commission priority first in your life

Before Jesus ascended to heaven after His resurrection, He instructed His disciples: ***"Go into all the world and preach the Good News to everyone, everywhere. Anyone who believes and is baptized will be saved. But anyone who refuses to believe will be condemned. These signs will accompany those who believe: They will cast out demons in my name, and they will speak new languages. They will be able to handle snakes with safety, and if they drink anything poisonous, it won't hurt them. They will be able to place their hands on the sick and heal them."***[141]

Okay, I do not have enough faith to handle snakes or drink poison, but I have been able to share the Good News and heal the sick. The people around you are in desperate need of the power of God for salvation and healing. May we who have received Christ never forget just how good the Good News is! The freedom we have in Christ is something we should never take for granted or abuse.

It's God's desire that none should perish and that all should repent (see 2 Peter 3:9). He uses us, His body, to love and reach out to those who are lost with this Good News. When we live by, trust, and obey God's will for our lives and are filled with His Spirit, we can live out this impossible life (with Him we can do all things). Then we will begin to experience life to its fullest with all the fruits God promises us, including peace, joy, patience, hope, and love.

No matter what gifts God has blessed you with, the most important is love. Put your love to the test of 1 Corinthians 13, one of the most beautiful portions of Scripture written by the apostle Paul as inspired by the Holy Spirit:

If I could speak all the languages of earth and of angels, but didn't love others, I would only be a noisy gong or a clanging cymbal. If I had the gift of prophecy, and if I understood all of God's secret plans and possessed all knowledge, and if I had

---

[141] Mark 16:15-18

such faith that I could move mountains, but didn't love others, I would be nothing. If I gave everything I have to the poor and even sacrificed my body, I could boast about it; but if I didn't love others, I would have gained nothing.

Love is patient and kind. Love is not jealous or boastful or proud or rude. It does not demand its own way. It is not irritable, and it keeps no record of being wronged. It does not rejoice about injustice but rejoices whenever the truth wins out. Love never gives up, never loses faith, is always hopeful, and endures through every circumstance.

Prophecy and speaking in unknown languages and special knowledge will become useless. But love will last forever! Now our knowledge is partial and incomplete, and even the gift of prophecy reveals only part of the whole picture! But when full understanding comes, these partial things will become useless.

When I was a child, I spoke and thought and reasoned as a child. But when I grew up, I put away childish things. Now we see things imperfectly as in a cloudy mirror, but then we will see everything with perfect clarity. All that I know now is partial and incomplete, but then I will know everything completely, just as God now knows me completely.

Three things will last forever—faith, hope, and love—and the greatest of these is love.[142]

3.5 Are You Well-acquainted with God?

Even if you have been in a relationship with God for years, you may not be experiencing the sense of freedom, peace, and joy described in this chapter. While it is true that we go through dry periods for a short time or a trial of our faith, the fruits of a life of

---

[142] 1 Corinthians 13:1-13

faith describe what the ordinary believer can and should expect to experience most of his or her life. If this isn't the norm for you, you should at least feel that you are moving in the right direction, increasingly seeing life from God's perspective and reacting to life's circumstances with this perspective in mind. If you want more freedom, peace, and joy, ask yourself some hard questions:

1. Have I abandoned my self, my ego?

2. Have I immersed myself in God, and am I experiencing the liberty, joy, and peace that come with this relationship?

3. Am I approaching life, people, and God meekly, with a soft heart, or am I proud, stubborn, defensive, or competitive?

4. Do I seek to live in obedience to God, doing things His way instead of my own—in my relationships, my career, with my money, and in all areas of life?

5. Are there areas of my life or heart that I hold back from God, areas of wrongdoing that I refuse to relinquish?

6. Are there things that I do in life, in an attempt to protect or comfort myself, that I shouldn't be doing, and instead should I be looking to God for that comfort or protection?

7. Have I surrendered the people in my life to God, or am I trying to control them, protect them from life, gain their approval, or constantly criticize them?

8. Are there things in God's Word that I am reluctant to believe or that I reject?

9. Do I really meditate on God's Word? Do I bring everything to Him in prayer and put aside my ego to learn from and love other believers?

10. Is there someone I have not yet forgiven? Do I need to apologize to someone for hurtful words or actions?

11. Am I spending time daily in God's Word? (If not, think back to when you first fell in love with God and renew your efforts to know and follow Him. Then, God's Word will be describing you when it says, *"Though you have not seen him, you love him; and even though you do not see him now, you believe in him and are filled with an inexpressible and glorious joy."*[143])

12. Am I sharing the Good News with my friends, family, and neighbors? (If not, why not?)

---

[143] 1 Peter 1:8

CHAPTER 4
Thriving in Your Body

4.1 Though Life Is Short (on this Earth), it can Still Be Good!

Case 1: Sixty year-old woman with moderately high blood pressure (150/90). No other health problems other than occasional headaches. Her doctor recommended high blood pressure medication, but she refused, preferring a more natural approach. My prescription, based on her signs and symptoms, was a combination of calcium and magnesium: 500 mg of calcium, 250 mg of magnesium taken in divided doses during the day and at bedtime. I also prescribed walking for 20 minutes four times per week. The only dietary changes I recommended were to decrease red meat intake, increase vegetable intake, and reduce coffee to an occasional cup. After three months of following this program, her blood pressure returned to normal.

This lovely woman happens to be my mother, and I'm happy to report (thanks to my sister's persistence and encouragement) that Mom has stuck to walking an average of five days per week for close to an hour each time. Although she has not been as consistent with her supplement routine, the walking has paid dividends. Not only has her blood pressure stabilized, but Mom has also lost weight and feels 20 years younger than she did before. I am proud of you, Mom!

Case 2: Fifty-three year-old woman with chronic fatigue syndrome and fibromyalgia. For several years, J had been suffering from severe chemical and environmental allergies. She had lost her voice and rarely left her house. By the time I met her, she had begun some natural products that had given her a glimmer of hope. She was on a mineral formula, chlorella, and an adrenal support product. She was now able to speak in a quiet, hoarse voice, and the pain from the fibromyalgia had been slightly reduced.

I tested her for food sensitivities and she was reacting to almost everything, so I put her on a restrictive diet initially. Brown rice, steamed vegetables, chicken, and fish were the foundation of her diet. I started her on low doses of an antifungal product containing rosemary and thyme oil, grapefruit seed extract, pau d'arco, and a few other ingredients. I later added vitamin C with bioflavinoids and IP6 (inositol hexaphosphate), both of which are known to enhance levels of the body's own natural killer cells. (Cells that help the body fight off abnormal cells and pathogens.) After a few months, she was able to go outside again, her voice was returning to full strength, and she began to talk about the possibilities of going back to work. As her body becomes stronger and with the addition of digestive enzymes, she should be able to tolerate adding the foods she was allergic to, at least on a rotational basis. NAET (Dr. Nambudripad's Allergy Elimination Technique) would also be useful in helping this individual tolerate foods better. I must acknowledge, however, that I have made many modifications to the NAET treatment and protocol, and I cannot guarantee the same results in other cases. In fact, if you follow all the steps in this chapter and book to improve your health and restore your mind, your allergies and sensitivities may be eliminated altogether without any treatment.

Case 3: Fourteen year-old with Crohn's disease with bleeding and extended abdomen and weight gain from prednisone. By the time she saw me her parents were overwhelmed with the side effects from the prednisone, and their daughter was also suffering from severe headaches. We prayed for a complete healing and wisdom in how I treated her. My testing revealed a sensitivity to eggs, yeast, and food additives. She also had an underlying dysbiosis (unhealthy intestinal flora—see Disease Model in Section 4.5).

I first put her on a treatment plan of colloidal silver to help kill some of the harmful bacteria, some Esberitox (echinacea, baptisia, and thuja) to boost her immune system, and had her avoid the food sensitivities for six weeks. Her symptoms began to improve over the next month, but the headaches were not getting better. Next I put her on a regimen of nux vomica homeopathic formula, began allergy treatment, and put her on some probiotics. Several months later she has had no more recurring episodes of her Crohn's symptoms and has had very few headaches. The only supplements she is currently taking on a regular basis are the probiotics and Esberitox in small doses.

Case 4: Forty-nine year-old women with chronic tremors, headaches, cough, ringing in ears, leg aches, sleep issues, sore throat, and fatigue. The most aggravating symptom: the tremors began after she was prescribed Synthroid for a low thyroid condition. When I first saw her almost three years ago, she was pacing in my office, unable to sit, and often crying uncontrollably. After much nutritional support, herbal support, adrenal support, changes in thyroid medication, candida treatment, and regular acupuncture treatments, this client has been able to live a somewhat normal life, but many of the underlying symptoms continue to persist at a lower level. Hair analysis and urine analysis with a chelator revealed mercury toxicity. A more recent genetic testing revealed slight errors in her DNA known as SNP's (single nucleotide polymorphisms)

that affected her ability to detoxify and handle oxidative stress. (For more information on these tests and others, go to www.drdyler.com.)

After many tests, many different mercury detoxification products, many herbal supplements, and a lot of prayer, this client has made further improvements, but she still has persistent low-grade symptoms. This journey towards health is not always easy, and some people may never be fully healed on this side of heaven. One thing is for sure though: my client has grown and matured spiritually through this process, and she has begun to lean on God daily for strength, direction, and peace. This can be a gift of illness, and the one who develops gratitude even in the midst of infirmity is one whom the Lord can use mightily.

Case 5: A physician colleague with whom I have consulted to discuss his patients' situations called me about three years ago to ask for help. He was diagnosed with prostate cancer. Radiation therapy and possible surgical procedures had been recommended. Since prostate cancer is a slow-growing cancer, I recommended that he go on an aggressive nutritional protocol. If there was no improvement in his cancer markers in six months, then he should proceed with the more invasive treatments. He agreed and was open to my prayers as well.

I recommended that he take several products. The first was a prostate formula called Pros-Forte that contains saw palmetto, pygeum, zinc, selenium, copper, vitamin D, pumpkin seed, stinging nettles, and lycopene. This combination would typically be utilized for BPH (benign prostatic hypertrophy), but I felt it would be helpful in his case as well. Next I recommended reduced glutathione in a patented form called Recancostat. Reduced glutathione is important in detoxification as an antioxidant, and it has been shown to boost immunity. I recommended he take a product called Healthy Cells Prostate, which contains calcium d-glucarate, broccoli extract, green tea, maitake mushroom, and some additional selenium. Calcium d-glucarate supplies the body with glucaric acid, which is an important substance used in the liver to excrete estrogens and xenobiotics (toxins that can mimic estrogen). He was already taking proteolytic enzymes between meals (a common protocol to reduce inflammation and potentially break down tumors), fish oil, CoQ10, calcium and magnesium, L-carnitine, and an herbal vitamin supplement. I specifically had him avoid B vitamins as I have a suspicion they may support the growth of candida or cancer cells. (This is my own theory and needs to be validated scientifically.)

One of the other things that my colleague says has specifically benefited him as well is a protocol called the Master Cleanse—a drink consisting of water, maple syrup and cayenne pepper to replace food for certain number of days. He does this cleanse every two to three months for three to seven days. I do not have enough personal experience with this cleanse to endorse it nor am I a big fan of too much sugar intake — including maple syrup. I believe that a cleanse should involve protein and extra nutrients which are critical for detoxification.

Well, the good news is that my friend called last week to tell me the doctors could no longer find cancer cells almost three years later! They did say there were still a few suspicious looking cells, but they would not identify them as cancer cells. To my friend, this simply meant that he should stay the course a while longer until there are only completely normal, healthy cells. Praise the Lord!

Note: By no means are the suggestions in this book nor the success stories on the previous pages an encouragement to self-diagnose or to self-treat medical conditions. Always consult with your health care practitioner before making any changes or additions to your treatment. Health and mental problems can be life-threatening and need professional input to avoid further complications. The goal of this chapter is to better educate you on how your body works, how it breaks down, and how you can best prevent getting sick in the first place.

4.2 Prevention Is Better Than Cure

Most of the patients that I see are not gravely ill. Instead, they come with chronic but irritating complaints that interfere with their ability to feel good and do their best in life. Whether the symptoms are mild, moderate, or severe, the person is no longer able to thrive in the present moment. Often, these symptoms are avoidable. In fact, I believe that 90 percent of chronic health issues are preventable with simple dietary, nutritional, and exercise lifestyles listed in this chapter, combined with the spiritual and mental principles and laws that I've covered in the previous chapters. The poor dietary, lifestyle, and exercise choices you make today may seem inconsequential but over time can and do lead to life-threatening conditions. Statistics tell us that, without a change in direction, most North Americans will eventually die of conditions related to heart disease or cancer.

The good news is that you can feel better and be healthier by making wise lifestyle choices that bring about improved health and quality of life. Living God's way will enable you to make changes in your life that you've never been able to make before. Living and thinking His way dramatically reduces the negative effects of stress on your health and well-being. You can also seek God's wisdom for your particular health situation and follow the counsel that I and many other holistic health practitioners promote for prevention of disease and optimization of health. It is, of course, a lot easier to prevent illness and disease than it is to treat them, but nonetheless there are answers and potential solutions to most health problems, whether cancer or acne, through diet, nutrition, and most importantly prayer.

The recommendations I make in this section are not fads or trends, but fundamental health practices—supported by science or significant clinical testing. When it comes to actual nutritional products, I acknowledge that there can always be improved products or protocols based on further clinical data or new research insights. Therefore, I recommend that you continue to walk with me on this journey of wellness by reading updates and expanded information that will be posted on my Web site at www.drdyler.com. I am always open to new and better ways of improving health that are documented, researched, or simply clinically effective. There are numerous empty promises and individuals seeking to profit from you. In particular, searching the Internet for health information can confuse you, scare you, hurt you, or most often waste your money. As with all things, you must discern fact from fiction. Ninety percent of what you read may be true, but it's the 10 percent you need to be careful about. I feel it is my responsibility and privilege to lead my patients to optimal health by providing them with information that is accurate, helpful, and effective. If I make mistakes, I hope I will be quick to acknowledge them and even quicker to correct them and lead you in the right direction. Please pray that I will always be a man of integrity, honesty, and humility.

4.3 The Wellness Spectrum

A wide spectrum exists between a state of perfect health and a life-threatening condition (see the Wellness Spectrum Diagram on page 169). How we were raised as children often determines not only our position on the spectrum, but also the direction in which we are heading—toward disease or toward health. Patterns and habits from our childhood need to be examined and eliminated if they do not serve to move us in the direction of optimal health.

If you find yourself in the "dis-ease" portion of the spectrum, you may not have received a diagnosis of a disease, but you may be experiencing many symptoms, such as fatigue, PMS, indigestion, or headaches. At the "danger zone" point on the spectrum, a person has only enough energy to get by in life. There's no energy to live life fully and creatively. As a person continues down the spectrum, he or she will tend to be more depressed, experience more chronic symptoms and illnesses, and be on more medications. More body systems will suffer chronic inflammation, manifested as the "-itis" conditions: arthritis, dermatitis, sinusitis, bronchitis, colitis, and so forth. Continued degeneration brings serious diseases such as heart disease, adult-onset (type 2) diabetes, osteoporosis, fibromyalgia, chronic fatigue syndrome, and, worse yet, cancer and neurological disorders.

For too many people, becoming older has become synonymous with a downward slide on the spectrum, with the body slowly but surely deteriorating into chronic illness and disability. Instead, the maturing process should lead, in most cases, to a time when we reach our full potential mentally, spiritually, and emotionally. Despite the aging process, we should be physically fit, energetic, and healthy.

Some of us have diseases and disabilities over which we have no control, but even so there may be measures we can take to improve our health and sense of well-being within the context of these challenges. For most people, changes in lifestyle, improved nutrition, natural treatments, and preventative measures will be all that is necessary to move on this spectrum from mere survival to a state of optimal well-being. Many of you may have tried and failed to make these changes. By closely following the spiritual principles in the previous two chapters, you can have the power to take the life-changing steps to improve your physical health that are outlined in this chapter. You can make the foundational changes that will help you prevent future diseases. What's more, you can move beyond mere physical well-being to a point where you can truly say that you are thriving in mind, body, and spirit.

The Wellness Spectrum

Which direction are you headed on the Wellness Spectrum? Are you covering up symptoms with over-the-counter medications? Is your body trying to tell you something?

4.3 The Wellness Spectrum

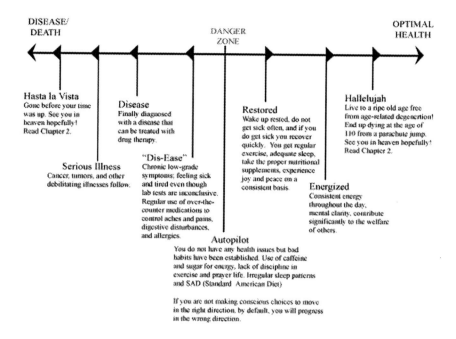

DISEASE/
DEATH

DANGER
ZONE

OPTIMAL
HEALTH

Hasta la Vista
Gone before your time
was up. See you in
heaven hopefully!
Read Chapter 2.

Disease
Finally diagnosed
with a disease that
can be treated with
drug therapy.

Restored
Wake up rested, do not
get sick often, and if you
do get sick you recover
quickly. You get regular
exercise, adequate sleep,
take the proper nutritional
supplements, experience
joy and peace on a
consistent basis.

Hallelujah
Live to a ripe old age free
from age-related degeneration!
End up dying at the age of
110 from a parachute jump.
See you in heaven hopefully!
Read Chapter 2.

Serious Illness
Cancer, tumors, and other
debilitating illnesses follow.

"Dis-Ease"
Chronic low-grade
symptoms; feeling sick
and tired even though
lab tests are inconclusive.
Regular use of over-the-
counter medications to
control aches and pains,
digestive disturbances,
and allergies.

Energized
Consistent energy
throughout the day,
mental clarity, contribute
significantly to the welfare
of others.

Autopilot
You do not have any health issues but bad
habits have been established. Use of caffeine
and sugar for energy, lack of discipline in
exercise and prayer life. Irregular sleep patterns
and SAD (Standard American Diet)

If you are not making conscious choices to move
in the right direction, by default, you will progress
in the wrong direction.

4.4 Physical Health from God's Perspective

Changing direction on the Wellness Spectrum to move toward optimum health can best be accomplished by bringing our physical health under God's direction. This process can have a profound impact on our enjoyment of life and on our ability to reach our full God-given potential and purposes. Of course God can and does use you no matter what your current health condition is like, but we can be much more effective in our ability to help others when we are feeling energized. To move in the right direction on the Wellness Spectrum, we must reduce stress, give our body adequate nutrition, support cleansing or detoxification, and most importantly gain wisdom and understanding from God's Word. We must not have any delusions about life, but rather make better choices every day to improve the quality of life while we are here. Always remember that life here on earth is short, but it can still be good.

When it comes to dietary choices what does the bible actually say? Should we be vegetarian? Drink wine? Consume goat's milk? Should we avoid pork and shellfish? One could make a case biblically for any of these dietary choices and they would not be wrong. One can also choose to eat or drink almost anything with God's blessings and they are right as well.

God gives us a lot of freedom in a lot of areas but it is important to remember moderation, common sense and respect for others in whatever dietary choices they make.

What is really important is that we do not confuse health practices with spirituality. Remember, the ego does not die easily and spiritual egoism is running rampant. For example, some people mistakenly think that if they abstain from eating meat and other substances, they will become more spiritually advanced. Following that erroneous line of thinking, the person who can live on one small bowl of plain, organic brown rice each day would represent the height of spiritual development! But God is clear on this point. Jesus spoke on this very matter:

"Listen and understand. What goes into a man's mouth does not make him 'unclean,' but what comes out of his mouth, that is what makes him 'unclean.'"[144]

He went on to explain:

"But the things that come out of the mouth come from the heart, and these make a man 'unclean.' For out of the heart come evil thoughts, murder, adultery, sexual immorality, theft, false testimony, slander."[145]

---

[144] Matthew 15:10-11
[145] Matthew 15:18-19

The apostle Paul wrote:

"Don't handle, don't eat, don't touch." Such rules are mere human teaching about things that are gone as soon as we use them. These rules may seem wise because they require strong devotion, humility, and severe bodily discipline. But they have no effect when it comes to conquering a person's evil thoughts and desires.[146]

Is this a green light to eat whatever we want, when we want, and how much we want of it? Of course not! God is warning us of religious attempts to reach Him through rituals and practices that will always fall short: wearing white, speaking softly, assuming various postures, abstaining from various foods and beverages, and so forth will never succeed. Why, we will do anything to become more spiritual except what God actually asks! We must examine our hearts and seek what He says pleases Him. The rewards are an abundant, joyful life and an intimate relationship with Him. *"Pay attention, my child, to what I say. Listen carefully. Don't lose sight of my words. Let them penetrate deep within your heart, for they bring life and radiant health to anyone who discovers their meaning."*[147]

Once again we are reminded of the interaction of mind, body, and spirit, and the importance of all of them. How can living in the awakened state lead to better health in the body as well as the mind? The Bible says in the New Testament, *"Physical exercise has some value, but spiritual exercise is much more important, for it promises a reward both in this life and the next."*[148] Keep this perspective in mind as we explore physical activities you can do to improve your health. Do not become obsessed or preoccupied with your health at the expense of spiritual pursuits. Having the right priorities will help you to improve your health, even bring radiant health, as you fall deeper and deeper in love

---

[146] Colossians 2:21-23 New Living Translation
[147] Proverbs 4:20-22 New Living Translation
[148] 1 Timothy 4:8 New Living Translation

with your Creator.

4.5 The Disease Model
To understand solutions, first understand causes

Stress, in its broadest sense, is the cause of most disease. I'm defining stress as anything that weakens the body or contributes to its degeneration. This includes toxins in the environment, traumas, poor diet, infections, allergies and sensitivities (food and environmental), genetic weaknesses, alcohol, drugs, emotional stress, lack of exercise, and structural imbalances. Even stress that is not based on reality, but is only perceived, can have negative consequences. An example of a real stress would be a vitamin deficiency that interferes with a person's immune system. An example of a perceived stress might be exaggerated fears that were created about the Y2K problem. Although the fear was out of proportion to reality, the body still reacts as if there were a very real danger. Fear, anger, resentment, worry, and sadness all can act as a constant physical stress.

Sometimes we are unaware that there is a source of stress. I have had clients who could not identify any obvious external stresses, yet their health was poor. They didn't realize that they had a major food allergy/sensitivity or an inherently weak organ system that was acting as a source of stress. When this was diagnosed and treated, they regained their health. For example, a patient might have weak liver function. If he accumulates small amounts of pesticides and environmental toxins, has wine with dinner each night, and frequently eats foods that he's allergic to, that may be enough to tip the scale toward disease. Someone else's body might be able to handle these same stresses. Our bodies have been created to handle a great deal of stress. In fact, some degree of stress not only is normal but also has the potential to foster maturity and spiritual growth. But the various stresses in our lives, real or perceived, within our control or beyond our control, set off biological changes, and these can have a cumulative effect. When the total stress load reaches a threshold level, vulnerability to disease is at its highest.

Imagine that you have a health checking account. As with any checking account, you add to the account each day as you "earn money": taking vitamins, eating well, exercising, sleeping well, and drinking plenty of water. You "withdraw money" from the account as you stress your body: smoking, eating junk food, drinking alcohol, and living a sedentary life. Make your own list of activities that build you up and ones that tear you down. Begin to get rid of or change your response to the stressful activities.

Genetics play a role, too. If you have received a large "inheritance," that is, a healthy constitution, you can live fairly recklessly for quite a while with very few consequences, at least physically. We've all seen people like this, who smoke, eat high fat foods, and don't exercise much, but seem to do fine. If that's you—stop playing Russian roulette with your life! You will eventually run out, no matter how big your inheritance was. Once you use up your inheritance, it is very difficult to restore, especially as you get older. Other people are born with a negative balance in their health checking account. They can't afford to cut any corners. Unless they are careful about nutrition, exercise, avoidance of environmental toxins, and other health factors, they will be vulnerable to disease.

Examine the Disease Model on page 177. Stress includes food allergies and sensitivities; emotional reactivity; electromagnetic radiation or frequencies that are harmful for our bodies (be careful with cell phones—they definitely contribute to car accidents and can potentially harm the brain); structural imbalances (see your chiropractor); environmental toxins; financial pressures; and, of course, poor lifestyle choices in general. Notice that no matter what the source of stress is, your brain (pituitary) sends signals to your adrenal glands, which produce stress hormones. Your adrenal glands are much like a car battery. When they get weak, your body starts to break down or doesn't start very well. Sleep disturbances often follow along with fatigue. The increased stress hormones and nervous system overdrive lead to poor digestion (inappropriate release of acid and decreased pancreatic enzymes), immune system deficiencies (decreased mucosal and microbial defenses) that set up a perfect environment for dysbiosis (pathogen overgrowth). This eventually leads to leaky gut syndrome that allows toxins and small food proteins to enter the blood stream, leading to allergies, chronic inflammation and decreases absorption of nutrients. The poor liver and lymphatic system get backed up with reactions to food proteins (antigen/antibody complexes) and a variety of toxins produced from the dysbiosis. When the liver can no longer adequately detoxify the body and when the immune system becomes depleted, toxins and infections can lead to a variety of disease processes. Toxins that are not safely excreted from the body can damage your kidneys and virtually every cell of your body. You will age faster and will be more prone to heart disease, cancer, stroke, Alzheimer's disease and a host of other serious illness. How symptoms manifest depend on your genetic susceptibilities and organ system weaknesses.

Even if you are fortunate enough not to develop a serious illness, you will begin to feel sick and tired if your total combined stress is too high. Individuals who have a vulnerable thyroid gland will usually gain weight and feel very sluggish. Individuals with vulnerable lymphatic systems will experience chronic sinusitis and post-nasal drip. Individuals with vulnerable nervous systems will feel dizzy and off balance. Many women will experience excess cramping and bloating with their period due to poor liver metabolism of hormones. Many individuals will suffer from joint pain and inflammation. Skin problems such as acne and rashes may plague you as well. After you review the Disease Model diagram, we will take a closer look at how the main organs and glands either contribute to our health or lead to disease depending on how effectively they are functioning.

Virtually everyone will (at some point) manifest symptoms related to experiencing the reality of this Disease Model because no one is immune to stress. An acute viral or bacterial infection may be enough to trigger this vicious cycle. A drug your doctor prescribes or an over-the-counter medication you use may be enough to create an extra burden on your liver that tips you over into chronic 'dis-ease.' Most of the time however, it is the total combined stress that becomes too high over an extended period of time. Be aware of the hidden stressors—especially environmental toxins, dental material incompatibilities and infection, artificial foods and preservatives, food allergies/sensitivities and electromagnetic radiation that can slowly but surely deplete your energy reserves. Since I emphasize food allergies/sensitivities as such a common source of stress throughout this chapter, I thought it would be best to address how to best identify them and treat them here.

Food allergies/sensitivities

Many people go to their allergist and do the standard skin allergy testing for a variety of environmental and food substances. These tests only pick up histamine mediated allergies and thus miss out on a whole host of other possible reactions. Most food allergies involve a delayed response antibody reaction. Small food proteins enter into the blood stream via leaky gut dysfunction (increased intestinal permeability) which should not normally be there. The body sees these as foreign substances (antigens) and produces different immune complexes to "fight" off the invader. These immune complexes (immunoglobulin antibodies) are usually of the IgG and IgM variety as opposed to the IgE (histamine) response that traditional allergists test for. That is why your test may come back normal for a food that you know you are reacting to. There are many doctors who run the IgG antibody panels, which are more accurate for food allergies, that are not anaphylactic in nature. i.e., a peanut allergy that triggers an asthma reaction or closing of the throat.

The only problem with the IgG panels is that antibodies can remain elevated for long periods of time even if your body is no longer acutely reacting to a food. For example, a cold or flu could trigger inflammatory reactions leading to leaky gut on a temporary basis and a host of food allergies could be triggered. That is why the old-wive's suggestion of chicken soup during a cold is wise because it avoids the most common foods that can cause or become an allergic reaction. Wheat, corn, soy, eggs, dairy are among the most common allergens.

Then there are food sensitivities—foods that give you a negative response within minutes or hours of eating them, which may not have anything to do with antibodies. Sugar, food colorings, MSG (monosodium glutamate), artificial flavorings, fruits and almost any food you can think of. Many health care practitioners incorporate applied kinesiology testing (muscle testing) or some electro dermal response testing device. Although these lack scientific evidence and can be variable between practitioners, I often find that the practitioners who are skilled in these practices get the best patient results.

Figuring food allergies/sensitivities out by yourself can be a very frustrating and tricky process. If you eliminate five but are missing a sixth unknown allergen your results may be very disappointing. I like to have clients avoid the foods that are suspected for four weeks before introducing them into the diet, one at a time, to see if they are problematic. A combination of diagnostic procedures may be necessary if you are not getting clinical success.

My goal with patients is always to get them to be able to eat all foods (not chemicals) and most of the time I am able to accomplish this by having clients follow the principles listed in the rest of this chapter. I also frequently utilize NAET (Dr. Nambudripad's Allergy Elimination Technique). See my website for more details. Occasionally for whatever reason, no matter what I do or recommend, a client is not able to tolerate a particular food and has to simply avoid it. I am happy to report that this is a rare occurrence and most people can eat all foods in moderation.

4.5: The Disease Model

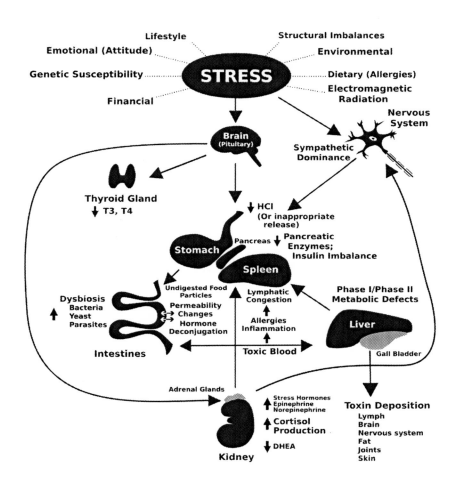

4.6 Understanding Your Organs and Glands

1. The Adrenal Glands

Some stress, the kind that stimulates the production of stress hormones, intensifies the effects of other types of stress, and pushes us down the Wellness Spectrum toward further degeneration. In our fast-paced culture, many people are experiencing the side effects of adrenal stress and fatigue: insomnia, fatigue, emotional edginess, feeling cold, dizziness, high or low blood pressure, poor recovery from illness, blood sugar swings and the resulting craving for sugar, poor memory, dependency on caffeine and other stimulants and the resulting low-level anxiety and poor coping mechanisms. Of course, many other conditions can trigger such events, but the adrenal glands are the batteries to your vehicle. When they are run down, everything else begins to break down.

Our first response to acute stress, such as a dog chasing us down the street, is alarm. In what is known as the fight-or-flight response, the brain causes the pituitary gland to send a chemical signal (the hormone ACTH) to the adrenal glands. The adrenal glands (which sit on the kidneys) then release adrenaline (epinephrine or norepinephrine). This normal response to acute stress increases our ability to either run from the dog or stand and fight the dog. The heart rate increases, glucose is released for immediate fuel needs, and blood flow increases to the muscles for increased activity and strength. We breathe faster to increase the supply of oxygen throughout the body. Many people can recognize the onset of an adrenaline surge, often felt as jitteriness and an uncomfortable feeling in the chest or stomach. In the second phase of the response, which is much longer lasting, cortisol and other hormones are released to keep energy up, and to increase sodium retention and blood pressure. This should be followed by a return to a relaxation state when the external stresses are gone.

Unfortunately, Americans go into the fight-or-flight response several times daily. They perceive situations as being potentially beyond their control or upsetting, and they experience psychological and emotional stress. This perception of a threat is enough to stimulate the release of stress hormones. A simple example of this would be the person who is caught in traffic. He has been on this route hundreds of times before and knows that the odds are high that traffic will move at a snail's pace at this time of day. Instead of popping in a tape of a good book or soothing music, he becomes angry and worries about being late to his evening activity. A car suddenly pulls out in front of him, and as he steps on the brake he feels a rush of adrenaline.

The potential for this type of stress and reaction is everywhere in our lives—in our relationships with family and co-workers, in our finances, and in how we react to a myriad of small and large life events. We perceive a threat, real, exaggerated, or imagined, and the fight-or-flight response is initiated. A flood of adrenaline is useful if you are a pedestrian who is about to be hit by a car. Your body is equipped by a rush of adrenaline to run faster than you ordinarily could. But brain cells can't tell the difference between stress caused by physical danger and stress caused by our reactions to a drop in the stock market or an irritable spouse. The same flood of stress hormones is released. This may leave us feeling tense, anxious, and nervous. Or, we may experience symptoms such as digestive problems (heartburn, nausea, and diarrhea), headaches, exhaustion, moodiness, depression, or have trouble falling asleep at night. Eating while under stress, or even eating when experiencing emotions such as anger or sadness, can cause improper digestion of food. Improperly digested food contributes to malnutrition, often leading to food sensitivities and increased metabolic waste for the body to handle.

The effects of chronic stress hormone exposure are amplified by other chronic stresses, such as inflammations caused by environmental toxins, unhealthy bacteria in the intestines, food allergies and blood sugar swings caused by eating too many simple carbohydrates. Over time, people may become unable to return to a fully relaxed state. Adrenaline levels remain high, even in the absence of stress. People may enter a maladaptive phase, where the cortisol level is elevated, DHEA (a precursor of sex hormones and corticosteroids) is decreased, and adrenaline is released inappropriately. In this phase, fatigue, anxiety symptoms, and sleep disturbances become the rule rather than the exception. Not only is the cortisol level elevated, but the normal fluctuation throughout the day is reversed. In a healthy person, cortisol levels are highest in the early morning and lowest by midnight. In the maladaptive phase, cortisol levels are low in the morning and elevated at night, thus interfering with sleep.

An elevated cortisol level has wide-ranging effects. It decreases the REM (rapid eye movement) phase of the sleep cycle, which decreases vitality and contributes to the breakdown of organ systems. It hampers the immune system. For example, it decreases activity of the natural killer cells that fight bacterial and viral infections, and even cancer. It lowers the amount of a substance (sIgA) that is the primary immune system defense mechanism for the mucus membranes, thus increasing susceptibility to upper respiratory infections and the growth of pathological organisms in the bowels. An elevated cortisol level increases calcium loss from the bones. It reduces insulin sensitivity, eventually causing higher blood sugar levels. Higher blood sugar levels can cause significant damage to various tissues in the body, as seen in diabetic patients. Elevated cortisol levels lead to the loss of lean body mass and its replacement with fat.

The final stage of adrenal fatigue occurs when the adrenal glands are so exhausted that they can no longer produce enough cortisol. The medical extreme of this is called Cushing's disease. Clinically, however, I see many patients that are still producing cortisol but inadequate amounts. Cortisol regulates inflammation and the immune system. Thus, in this stage of adrenal fatigue, there is much more autoimmune disease and skin and joint inflammation.

Adrenal Treatment

In terms of supporting and rebuilding the adrenal glands, a lot depends on your adrenal glands' current strength. I would recommend that you have your doctor run an adrenal salivary hormone profile to assess the current state of your adrenals. You can read more about this on my Web site, www.drdyler.com. You can order the test from the Web site and perform the test yourself.

Most of the time, the adrenal glands naturally start to improve when food allergies and sensitivities are avoided, nutritional deficiencies are corrected, a balance of complex carbohydrates, proteins, and fats are consumed, and digestion is improved. When the adrenal glands are depleted, stimulants like caffeine, ginseng, and rhodiola will give temporary benefits, but will eventually lead to further depletion, especially if you are not working on eliminating the underlying stresses in your life.

If your adrenal glands are mildly fatigued, the best strategy is short naps, regular exercise, and perhaps some extra vitamin C, B vitamins (B5 in particular), magnesium, and added salt. Most people with adrenal deficiency do well with some additional sodium because sodium levels become depleted with chronic adrenal stress.

Many products have glandular extracts from animals that contain the building blocks for helping to repair your adrenals. It is important that they are of high quality and used sparingly while you're working on the underlying stresses. Licorice root can be helpful but can also raise blood pressure in susceptible individuals and thus blood pressure needs to be monitored.

Moderate to severe adrenal fatigue should be treated in conjunction with a qualified health care practitioner, who can determine the state of the adrenal glands from a saliva test. Treatment with the adrenal hormones DHEA and cortisol may be necessary. And remember, treating or supporting the adrenal glands without reducing the underlying stresses is simply a Band-Aid!

2. The Intestines

Long-term effects from years of overproduction of stress hormones can include adrenal fatigue, food allergies, hypertension, adult-onset (type 2) diabetes, and a host of other illnesses, including autoimmune diseases, irritable bowel syndrome, and even frequent colds. Recurrent infections are common, caused by candida, parasites, and bacteria. Killing the organisms does not achieve a permanent cure, because the underlying conditions that support the disease have not been treated effectively. Stress can also cause the body to release insufficient amounts of digestive secretions such as pancreatic enzymes, or insufficient and inappropriate amounts of hydrochloric acid leading to heartburn. Without these critical digestive aids, some food decomposes in the intestines instead of actually being digested. Improperly digested food leads, in turn, to dysbiosis, the overgrowth of pathological bacteria, yeast, or parasites in the intestines. The presence of these organisms can strain the immune system and be the cause of many of the symptoms we experience. These organisms produce toxins, which make us feel sick and weak. Each time we consume sugar in our food or in alcoholic beverages, we provide a feast for these pathogens. The toxins they produce irritate and inflame the lining of the intestines. I have tried many different candida products over the years, but the one that I first used when I was in medical school, Phytostan, continues to be the most effective for this problem. Phytostan contains beta carotene, undecylenic acid, caprylic acid, glutamic acid, grapefruit seed extract, rosemary oil, and thyme oil. Oregano oil, colloidal silver, and garlic have also been helpful for many people suffering from candida and other microbial imbalances (dysbiosis)

Over time, dysbiosis can lead to a condition of increased intestinal permeability, sometimes referred to as leaky gut syndrome. Normally, the intestinal wall provides a barrier that allows some substances to pass into the bloodstream and prevents other, sometimes harmful substances from entering. In cases of leaky gut syndrome, inflammation of the intestinal wall creates an increase in permeability, so that some of the substances, which were previously prevented from entering the bloodstream, are now able to enter. Certain substances aggravate leaky gut syndrome, including alcohol, aspirin, improperly digested food, chemicals, and pesticides. Once leaky gut syndrome develops, the proteins in dairy (whey and casein), the gluten in grains, and the albumin in eggs can enter the bloodstream, causing systemic reactions (food allergies) that aggravate symptoms even further. As the immune system goes into overdrive, chronically reacting to these proteins, it eventually becomes depleted, leaving us vulnerable to other diseases. Once the permeability problem becomes advanced, viruses, bacteria, parasites, and candida are also able to penetrate the intestinal wall and affect the blood, the organ systems, and the nervous system.

I find that eliminating food allergies and sensitivities and killing off candida, pathological bacteria, and parasites is usually the best strategy for dealing with leaky gut syndrome. Stool analysis can determine the presence of these microbes. I frequently use a therapeutic trial with substances that are effective at killing off these pathogens. In Chinese medicine, this imbalance can often be determined by a thick or sticky tongue coating. This can indicate an overgrowth of candida, bacteria, or parasites. After killing off the bad bugs, replacing them with good strains of bacteria is critical to maintain intestinal health. Also helpful in the repair process are the amino acid l-glutamine, NAG (n-acetyl glucosamine), butyric acid, digestive enzymes, and vitamins A, C, and E.

3. The Liver

The liver is the organ primarily responsible for detoxifying the blood. Although it's a very hardy organ system, the liver is vulnerable to a constant source of toxins, food reactions, medications and infections.

In medical terms, there are two main detoxification phases in the liver. Phase I involves the P450 enzyme systems, which are responsible for initially metabolizing toxins and drugs and creating intermediate compounds that need to be further detoxified. That's where the phase II pathways are involved. In this phase the intermediate compounds are bound to substances, such as sulphur, amino acids, glutathione, and glucaric acid. Herbs such as milk thistle (silymarin) and dandelion root and food extracts, such as beet root and artichoke, can help with overall liver function.

When the body is nutritionally depleted and has been under stress, an extra burden is placed on the liver. This leads to a greater vulnerability to environmental toxins and our own metabolic waste, leading to increased oxidative stress—the same process that causes metal to rust damages cells in our bodies. When the liver is overwhelmed, the process of building new proteins to repair the body, activating thyroid hormones, regulating cholesterol, and providing glycogen for immediate fuel needs, becomes compromised. Any genetic predisposition for problems in specific areas of our bodies, whether it be your joints, lungs, nervous system, throat, sinuses, skin, or brain, will be aggravated when your liver cannot keep up with detoxification. In Chinese medicine, liver troubles will be associated with a tense, wiry pulse, and oftentimes the sides of the tongue will appear redder in color.

Proper liver function is critical for one's state of well-being and as you will read below—most people will benefit from occasional or more frequent liver support. My website www.drdyler.com will give you more details and insight to see if a liver detoxification protocol is right for you.

Are You Toxic?

In 1990, the Environmental Protection Agency conducted a study involving 1,377 individuals. One hundred percent of adipose (fat) tissue samples contained dioxin, dichlorobenzene, styrene, xylene, and ethyphenol. Seventy-six percent of the samples had the PCB benzene and a host of other chemicals. In another study, individuals who ate organic foods did not fare much better.

In 2004, the Ontario College of Family Physicians completed a review of available literature on the health effects of pesticide exposure. Highlights include:

- A leukemia study conducted in Montreal revealed that 40 percent of children had a specific genetic vulnerability to pesticides.
- A Swedish cancer study revealed that three to seven percent of non-Hodgkin's lymphomas were directly attributable to pesticide exposure.

You also may be burdened with chemical or toxin overload and by heavy metals such as mercury, lead, cadmium, and aluminum, which can wreak havoc on your endocrine and nervous systems. Please go to my Web site (www.drdyler.com) to view sources of heavy metals and the possible symptoms they cause. Treatment for heavy metals is complex and should be done under the supervision of a qualified health care practitioner to prevent further damage to the nervous system, kidneys, and adrenal glands. Oftentimes, gentle detoxification with diet and herbs, along with exercising, saunas, and additional nutritional support can help to reduce the toxic burden safely over time.

In conclusion, we all need to detoxify, but safely.

4. The Spleen/Lymphatic System

The spleen is actually comprised of two systems: a white pulp immune system that generates antibodies to attack circulating foreign substances (antigens), and a red pulp reticuloendothelial system that acts like a big mop cleaning up debris (phagocytes and granulocytes). The immune system produces and matures B and T lymphocytes and plasma cells that help the body fight off infection. If you suffer from recurrent colds, sinus infections, and post-nasal drip, your spleen/lympathic system is overwhelmed by one or more of the following: food allergies and sensitivities, metabolic wastes, toxins generated from fungal, bacterial, parasitic, or viral infections, or environmental poisons. Identifying food allergies and sensitivities is critical in helping support a healthy lymphatic system as is supporting the immune system and assisting colon and liver detoxification.

Exercise and massage greatly enhance lymphatic circulation, and certain herbs like echinacea, burdock root, dandelion root, and red clover can be very helpful as well. From the perspective of Chinese medicine, the spleen is somewhat equivalent to the pancreas' digestive function in Western medicine. In other words, digestive enzymes are critical to ensure that food substances are properly digested and assimilated. When your spleen (pancreas) is weak, your tongue will tend to be swollen and have what appears to be teeth indentations on the sides. Taking digestive enzymes with meals can be an important step to cleanse the lymphatic system and assist the immune system.

5. The Thyroid Gland

The thyroid gland is responsible for healthy metabolism; when it's operating sub-optimally, weight gain and sluggishness usually follow. When many of my clients initially come to see me, they are either taking thyroid medication or in need of some kind of thyroid support.

The adrenal glands and the thyroid work hand in hand to help maintain the ideal metabolism for burning calories and eliminating cellular wastes. When either of these glands becomes depleted, it puts an extra burden on the other gland to perform more rigorously. The adrenal gland is most affected by stress whereas the thyroid gland is more vulnerable to toxins such as heavy metals and substances like chlorine, fluorine, and bromine. Many people on low sodium diets often become depleted in iodine, which is extremely important for thyroid function. Worse yet, many individuals no longer use iodized salt, which is where most North Americans get their iodine. Regardless of the cause of a sub-optimal thyroid function, poor metabolism leads to even more accumulation of toxins in the body, and chronic illness is sure to follow.

Diagnosis of low thyroid function, called hypothyroidism, should include blood tests for levels of free T3, T4, and TSH. Many people suffer from chronic low-grade thyroid function, which may or may not show up on blood tests because normal ranges of thyroid hormone levels are so wide. A low body temperature is one of the possible indicators of low thyroid function. (See the section on Weight Loss in 4.12, for specifics on the home test you can do.)

If thyroid hormone replacement treatment is necessary, ask your doctor about Armour Thyroid, which has a complete array of thyroid hormones including calcitonin. Many people seem to do well on synthetic thyroid replacement, but others hit a wall and their progress stalls. If you are officially diagnosed with low thyroid, ask your doctor to run a test to see if you have thyroid antibodies—*i.e.,* autoimmunity to your own thyroid. If you do, you most likely have low cortisol levels, suffer from other allergies, and could potentially have heavy metal toxicity, contributing to a dysfunctional immune system. Less common and more difficult to treat is an excess thyroid state, called hyperthyroidism. The cause of this is somewhat of a mystery, but is most likely related to genetic predispositions, nervous system overdrive and sensitivity to iodine. Excess thyroid can cause a fast heart rate and severe anxiety, and most often needs serious medical intervention, such as radioactive iodine to shut down the thyroid or surgical removal of the thyroid gland. If you follow the principles in this book and this section in particular, both hypothyroidism and hyperthyroidism can likely be avoided. As I stated previously, prevention is always better than looking for a cure and stress reduction can do wonders.

Supportive nutritional products for low thyroid function include iodine, the amino acid tyrosine, which is a precursor to thyroid hormones, and perhaps some animal glandular extracts, much like the ones used in many adrenal support products. Often nutritional support products with the ingredients listed above can lessen your need or dependence on thyroid prescriptions, especially if underlying toxicity issues, such as heavy metals, are addressed.

Treating the thyroid can be complicated and is best done under qualified medical supervision.

4.7 Stress and Health: A Self-assessment Test

Studies show that when people do poorly on stress questionnaires, they have a significantly higher than average chance of experiencing a major illness in the following year. The relationship between stress and physical health is a two-way street: physical health affects how well we tolerate stress and cope with it; chronic stress, in turn, damages our physical health.

187

Some stress tests measure how much stress is in your life; for example, has a family member died recently, or have you lost your job? While results of these tests do correlate with future health, a much more important question, regardless of the amount of stress you have, is, "How is your body and mind handling the stress in your life?"

Use this test to assess your current level of stress-related symptoms. Place a number at each hyphen below, based on how often you experience that symptom. Then add up the numbers to calculate your symptom level.

0 = Never
1 = Occasionally
2 = Frequently
3 = Daily or almost every day

During the past month, have you experienced?

EMOTIONS
__Depression
__Dreading the next day
__Feeling like life is out of control
__Feeling pessimistic or helpless
__Feeling stressed when doorbell or phone rings
__Feeling emotionally exhausted
__Feeling restless
__Feelings of failure
__Feelings of anger
__Having imaginary "arguments" all day with people
__Impatience
__Irritability
__Nervousness, anxiety, or worry

PHYSICAL SYMPTOMS
__Allergies

__Back pain
__Biting or chewing nails
__Butterflies in stomach
__Diarrhea or constipation
__Dry mouth
__Fatigue unrelated to lack of sleep
__Frequent heartburn
__Headaches
__Increased sweating
__Infections, including colds and flu
__Insomnia
__Jaw-clenching
__Lack of energy
__Loss of appetite
__Muscle tension, especially in neck and shoulders
__Nausea unrelated to specific illness
__Pounding heartbeat
__Rapid breathing
__Rapid or irregular heartbeat
__Rashes or hives
__Sexual problems
__Stomach discomfort
__Tics or twitches
__Tightness in chest

BEHAVIORS
__Calling in "sick" to work
__Crying, teary-eyed
__Difficulty concentrating, even when there are no distractions
__Drinking too much alcohol
__Easily startled
__Eating a lot of junk food
__Emotional outbursts
__Excessive food intake
__Focusing on critical thoughts about others
__Increased cigarette smoking

__Increased use of medication
__More forgetful than usual
__Neglecting your closest relationships
__Overreacting to small incidents
__Overspending or overly concerned with finances
__Procrastination about important tasks
__Using illegal drugs
__Watching too much television

0-20 Symptom level is better than average

21-40 Symptom level is average. Keep in mind, however, that the average person in our modern world is experiencing a great deal of stress, which is taking its toll on physical health. "Average," unfortunately, is not the same as "healthy." Follow the recommendations in this book to avoid problems in the future.

41-50 Symptom level is higher than average. Make changes and consider getting help from your physician, friends, etc. If you continue on your current path, you may develop stress-related disease within the next year.

51+ Symptom level is very high. Consult with a physician as soon as possible, and devote yourself to making the changes in this book. Like any profession there are good and bad doctors. Shop around for and better yet get a referral from a friend for a qualified and effective naturopath, chiropractor, acupuncturist, or medical doctor trained in integrative medicine. (Integrative medicine incorporates modern medicine with traditional or alternative medicine.)

Regardless of your total score, you should address any 3's on the list as indicative of a potentially serious problem.

If you have conditions/symptoms such as high blood pressure, migraines, depression, autoimmune diseases, heart arrhythmia, colitis, or chronic fatigue, your symptom level should automatically be considered "very high" regardless of your test score.

If you follow the recommendations in this book, including the specific changes suggested in this chapter, take the test again in three months, and again in six months, to see if your score is moving in the right direction. You'll be amazed by the results.

4.8 Breaking Out of the Stress/Disease Cycle

You can break out of this cycle of stress and disease! I did! It's possible to completely change direction on the spectrum of health and well-being described at the beginning of this chapter. We must take three steps, steps that will lead not only to better health, but also to greater happiness.

STEP ONE: Take hold of God's power to make the changes you've never been able to make in the past.

Our main problem usually isn't lack of information, is it? Virtually everyone knows that we should eat less fat and sugar, drink lots of water, get adequate sleep, and exercise regularly. Our main problem related to health is making changes and sticking with them. Most people set unrealistic goals and thus set themselves up for failure. Good habits take time to develop; perfectionism robs you of joy in the healing process, which takes time.

Some of us don't make healthful changes simply because we haven't taken the steps to discipline ourselves. In this case, simple measures, such as teaming up with another person, taking a class, or making charts and checklists, combined with prayer, are usually all that we need to help us succeed. But many of us have repeatedly struggled to make changes and failed each time. Help is available! For those who know Him, God offers life-changing, miraculous help every day. He empowers us to do what we've never been able to do before. He sometimes offers this help in response to one simple prayer, in the form of a sudden miracle. Pray for one! Often, He offers this help only if we surrender to

Him daily, minute by minute. In fact, He may allow these challenges in our lives to teach us certain lessons, become dependent on Him, and grow closer to Him. However it happens, He is able and pleased to help you.

STEP TWO: Be patient!

Every day, physicians see patients who would like a quick fix, a magic bullet. They come with diseases and conditions that they have spent a lifetime developing, yet they want a pill or treatment that will cure the problem immediately. Patients also want miraculous programs: six weeks to health, weight-loss programs based on everything from grapefruit to exotic herbs, fitness regimens built on complicated cross-training schedules. Unfortunately, for most people, virtually all of these programs eventually fail. What works? What is the Ultimate Weight-loss Fitness Anti-aging Beauty Virility Optimal Health Program? The most successful program is to permanently incorporate into our lives the simple things that God has supplied for our good health.

I use the word "permanently" because, as we all know, temporary measures simply don't lead to lasting results. Studies have repeatedly proven that diets (short-term changes in what you eat) do not work. Statements such as "I will lower my intake of saturated fat until I lose 20 pounds" and "I will cut down on stressful activities until I feel calmer" generally haven't led to success in the past, have they? Soon after we return to our normal nutrition and activity levels, the associated problems return. Take baby steps when you are beginning to incorporate healthful lifestyle practices so that you can make them permanent.

Making God our first priority will lead to a balanced mind and healthy emotions, which in turn will help us to stay on that narrow road to optimal health. We must always try to get to the root cause of our problems so that we are not using Band-Aids (medications) to cover up our symptoms. That is not to say that medications do not have a place, but rather always seek to gain an understanding of the reasons our bodies are out of balance. Many doctors are quick to prescribe drugs even when simple changes can make a difference. For example, government-funded studies have now shown that changing your diet to include lots of fruits and vegetables, and some dairy products, while simultaneously reducing fat intake, will be as effective at lowering blood pressure as taking medication. I don't advocate stopping your medication, but following the steps I've listed later in this chapter may lower your blood pressure enough to merit a discussion with your physician about reducing or eliminating your medication. This holds true for adult-onset diabetes, digestive problems, obesity, depression, insomnia, and hundreds of other conditions and symptoms.

STEP THREE: Get educated and incorporate simple, fundamental, researched, natural medicine practices.

All too often, people think of "natural medicine" as pills, herbs, and special supplements to buy. But natural medicine, at its heart, is comprised of measures that God has provided: drinking plenty of water, getting enough sleep, walking, getting enough vitamins, minerals, and fiber, and so forth. I've watched in frustration over the years as some patients look for that magic pill to fix what simple dietary and lifestyle changes would cure. Really drink those eight glasses of water a day. Go for a walk every day, pray, and meditate on God's Word daily. Before buying expensive, exotic, nutritional products, make sure that you incorporate these basic dietary, lifestyle and nutritional principles that will surely improve your quality of life.

4.9 Proper Nutrition

Some of these suggestions may sound basic to you, but it's amazing how many people (including myself) get off track. These fundamental dietary, nutritional, and lifestyle suggestions will help you to get on the right track by assisting your body to do what it already is made to do—heal!

• **Enjoy your food—chew, chew, chew.** It's easy in our fast-paced lives to eat on the run and not truly enjoy our food. If possible, at least one meal each day should be a sit-down meal with loved ones where there is conversation and enjoyment of the food. Turn off the TV and actually talk to your loved ones and friends! Setting a beautiful table and having a vase with fresh flowers can add to the relaxing environment.

Chewing food helps you to produce enzymes that will help you to assimilate and get the nutrients from the food you are eating.

Pray and give thanks for every meal. You can do it silently or out loud with family and friends.

God has created an enormous array of wonderful, delicious natural foods for your health and enjoyment. The Standard American Diet (notice the acronym SAD—that's what it is) is heavy in salt, fat, sugar, pesticides, artificial colors, flavors, and preservatives. Processed foods have been stripped of so much of their nutritional value, though a few synthetic vitamins may be thrown back in, that they shouldn't even be categorized as "food." For example, frozen casseroles (even ones that are supposedly "leaner" than other frozen meals—they're usually just smaller!), store-bought cookies and crackers, canned soups, rice mixes, and many other processed foods are loaded with sodium, hydrogenated fats, and other potentially harmful ingredients. Check the labels carefully.

Artificial sweeteners, even the ones that have not yet been identified as dangerous, should be reduced or avoided altogether.

Minimize the use of the microwave—who knows how many nutrients the microwave kills? Although I have not seen any scientific evidence about this, there have been reports that plants do not grow well when given water that has been microwaved. Nothing like a stove-cooked meal anyway!

• **Strive for balance.** The healthiest diet for most people is 40 percent complex carbohydrates, 30 percent protein, and 30 percent fat. Moderation in all things, except for your pursuit of God, is a good general rule. I promote the 80/20 rule. If you're healthy and eating healthily 80 percent of the time, you can occasionally eat a small dessert, muffin, cookies, an occasional soda pop, hot dog, a bag of chips, or, yes, even a McDonald's meal! Just don't abuse this rule. It means that out of 10 meals, you could have two "junk" or "fast-food" items. This rule applies only if you are generally healthy, exercising, and taking some good quality supplements. If you are struggling with your health, are overweight, and are not exercising routinely, I would recommend the 90/10 rule. If you are very ill or are a purist, then the 99/1 rule would apply.

Healthy snacks should begin to replace the junk food. And remember, chocolate is not a vegetable. (Okay, maybe dark chocolate comes close!) Choose to snack on celery sticks, carrot sticks, nuts and seeds, fresh fruits, whole grain breads and crackers, a variety of cheeses, and a wide range of healthy snacks available at your local health food store. Better yet, bake your own bread and experiment with new healthy snack recipes.

• **Move toward healthier fats.** Shift the emphasis in your diet from saturated fats to monounsaturated fats (like olive oil), omega-3 fats (found in flaxseed, salmon, tuna, and anchovies), and polyunsaturated fats (found in grape seed, sunflower, safflower, corn, flax, and sesame oil). Most people in North America are getting enough omega-6 oils but are deficient in omega-3s. Since a lot of deep water fish is contaminated with mercury, an omega-3 supplement is a must. I would still recommend eating deep-water fish once a week as an overall health plan and a way to add variety to your diet, but this will not satisfy the need for extra omega-3s. Salmon (wild, not farm-raised) is probably one of your safer choices a long with sardines. Tuna, although popular, should be limited to once a week due to mercury concerns. Making your own salad dressings with a mixture of olive oil and flax oil combined with balsamic vinegar or lemon and a touch of sea salt is a great health practice. Adding some fresh nuts and seeds can also add to the balance of omega-6 oils needed in the diet.

Eliminate trans fats, such as partially hydrogenated soybean oil and margarine—a few margarines are labeled free of trans fats, but I still prefer butter. Saturated fats should be limited to less than 10 percent of your daily calorie intake; I'd recommend much less, if possible. Limit fried foods as much as possible. Frying oils creates a significant amount of free radicals (unstable compounds) which can damage your body. Stir frying with olive oil or sesame oil is generally considered a healthy practice and does limited damage to the oils. Grape seed oil is probably the best oil for high temperature cooking—it's been shown in some smaller studies to raise the good HDL cholesterol and lower the LDL cholesterol. Grape seed oil is high in naturally occurring antioxidants. It would be worth your while tracking down this oil if you like frying or deep-frying your foods. Peanut oil is also good for high heats. Adding garlic, ginger, and other spices to your stir fry can further protect the oils by their additional antioxidant content. Reusing oils, which is the practice of many fast-food restaurants, produces an extremely high level of free radicals.

Learn to cook healthful and creative meals at home as much as possible.

• **Stick with low-fat protein.** Most of our protein should come from low-fat sources, including skinless chicken, lean meat, fish, tofu, beans, soy products, and low-fat cheese. Some of us can also afford to eat eggs occasionally, as well as moderate to high fat protein sources.

• **Drink for health.** Drink at least two quarts (eight cups) of water daily. As much as possible, reduce colas, fruit juices, and coffee. Many people can tolerate a cup or two of coffee a day, but others are sensitive to caffeine and should eliminate it completely. Caffeine in even moderate amounts can increase feelings of stress and anxiety. If you feel edgy after a cup of coffee, it has more caffeine than your body can handle. Decaffeinated coffee and tea often uses many chemicals in the decaffeination process and can be more harmful then caffeine itself.

Make sure that your water is from a pure source. Home filters can become contaminated quickly so make sure to change them frequently. To avoid diluting your digestive juices, minimize you intake of water at your main meals. Adequate hydration is important to health. Simply drinking more water, for example, helps prevent kidney stones, bladder cancer, and dry eyes. Mild dehydration can contribute to dry, itchy skin, headaches, constipation, and sluggishness, among other symptoms.

Caffeinated beverages are actually dehydrating and shouldn't be counted as part of your eight glasses of water per day. An occasional six-ounce glass of freshly squeezed orange juice or 100 percent Concord grape juice is acceptable, but try to avoid drinks with added sugar or corn syrup. Tomato juice is also beneficial because it contains a powerful antioxidant called lycopene, which helps protect against prostate cancer. Carrot juice is high in beta-carotene, but contains too much natural sugar and should be consumed only occasionally. Fresh grapefruit juice has many health benefits but must be avoided if you are on certain medications. Some of the water you drink can be herbal tea; green tea in particular has a lot of antioxidants.

• **Try one new healthy food each week.** A healthy diet doesn't have to be boring. Explore ethnic grocery stores and natural food stores. Have you ever had tofu, tempeh, quinoa, kiwi or mango fruit, balsamic vinegar, or garbanzo beans? I am blessed that my wife is Iranian as I have enjoyed many wonderful Persian foods and recipes. One of my favorites is called fesen jun, which is made from ground walnuts in pomegranate syrup with lean chicken. I'm getting hungry just thinking about it!

Check www.drdyler.com for recipes that are unique, healthy, and culturally diverse. That small group you've developed as a support network should plan some social gatherings to try out new recipes. My wife will be coordinating many of these suggestions on my Web site. I hope we can join you for dinner, discussion, and prayer!

• **Increase the fiber in your diet.** Try to eat 25 to 35 grams a day or more. Beans, whole grain breads (the ingredient list should start with 100 percent whole wheat), and oats are good sources, as are many fruits and vegetables. A low-fiber diet is associated with higher rates of many diseases. Following the other advice in this nutrition section will automatically provide you with enough fiber so that you won't need to count grams of fiber religiously. Freshly ground flaxseed, a good source of fatty acids and fiber, can be added to your daily diet.

• **Add more vegetables (and fruits) to your diet.** As a rule, most people do not get enough fruits and vegetables in their diet.

The American Cancer Society continues to increase the number of servings of fruits and vegetables people need to help prevent cancer. Currently the recommendation is for nine servings daily! How many servings are you currently getting?

I am a little more cautious with recommending increasing fruit consumption because so many people suffer from candida problems (fungi) or other microbes that feed on sugar. Many people who also suffer from adrenal fatigue cannot afford to have any swings in their blood sugar levels. If you do not have these problems, then by all means eat your fruit!

Washing fruits and vegetables with water is not sufficient to remove dangerous pesticides. If you are not buying all organic produce (and my wife and I do not, because of the cost), then put your fruits and vegetables in a tub of water with a few drops of dish soap (or other product for washing pesticides off of fresh produce). Wash gently by hand and rinse thoroughly.

Keeping your refrigerator stocked with ready-to-eat fruits and vegetables will help you avoid unhealthy snacks. Fruits and vegetables are rich in flavinoids, vitamins, minerals, and other important nutrients. The fiber found in fruits and vegetables will help with weight loss, high blood pressure, constipation, and the prevention of many diseases. Cruciferous vegetables such as broccoli, cauliflower, brussel sprouts, and cabbage are particularly high in compounds that help to detoxify your body. In general, raw fruits should be eaten about a half hour before meals or an hour afterward to avoid digestive problems (gas, bloating, and indigestion).

Planting a garden or a few pots of vegetables can be both therapeutic and fun. If you have children get them involved as well.

• **Eat a handful of nuts daily.** Minimize your intake of salted, oil-roasted nuts. Raw or dry roasted (better for individuals with poor digestion) almonds, pistachios, walnuts, and peanuts are great sources of nutrition. Most nuts are high in fat and calories, so use them sparingly if you are overweight, especially if you suspect you won't be able to stop with only two tablespoons. But eating the recommended amount of nuts is associated with a significantly lower rate of heart disease.

4.10 Exercise Now or Pay the Price Later

Exercise decreases the risk of heart disease, osteoporosis, diabetes, and many other conditions. In fact, regular exercise can reduce the risk of a heart attack by as much as 50 percent. Studies have also shown that walking reduces depression and increases the level of endorphins, the brain chemicals that give us a feeling of well-being and calmness. Endorphins are a sort of natural, mild morphine. Exercise helps our bodies to detoxify more efficiently and helps our adrenal glands to become stronger. I have found that my body can tolerate carbohydrates much more efficiently when I am exercising on a regular basis.

• **Walk!** If you aren't in shape, work up slowly to 30 to 60 minutes five or more times a week. If all you can manage in the first week is a walk to the end of the block and back, start there! Do it every day. You'll be amazed at how quickly you are able to increase the distance and speed of your walk. Get tapes of music or books to listen to while you walk, or tapes of the Bible. Use the time to meditate on God's Word, to pray, and to sing songs of praise from your soul. Talking things over with God while you're walking can be very productive and stress reducing. Pay attention to the beauty of God's creation. Everything from a bird singing to blossoms on a tree to the heavens filled with stars testify of God's creativity and splendor.

• **Take it easy.** Extreme plans usually don't last long. Studies show that people who exercise in the morning are more likely to stick with their program.

• **Have a backup plan.** Sometimes we don't have the time, energy, or motivation to walk for 30 to 60 minutes. Skipping a couple of days can easily lead to a week without exercise, and before we know it we've completely abandoned our exercise program. Two things will help. First, have a backup plan. On rainy days, for example, be prepared to ride a stationary bicycle, use a treadmill, do some stretching, or lift some dumbbells in the comfort of your home. Or have a regular date to walk with a friend once a week at the mall. Second, make sure you do something every day. If you're short on time or don't feel great, walk for 10 minutes instead of 45. Often, once we get moving, we're able to do more than we thought possible.

• **Make exercise enjoyable!** Regularly get other forms of exercise, preferably activities you enjoy. You might set a goal to do one activity a week that involves enjoyable exercise: dancing, hiking, canoeing, or swimming, for example. Gardening or other yard work can build health and has even been shown to promote healthy bones in women over 50 years of age. There are two kinds of exercises that promote strong bones. The first is weight-bearing exercise, such as walking, jumping, running, playing tennis, and similar activities that place stress on legs and hips. Ideally, this should be done for about half an hour, five days a week. The second kind is weight-lifting or strength-training. These types of exercises also place a stress on bones, which stimulates new bone growth. Ideally, you should strive for two or three strength-training sessions a week. In one study at Tufts University, researchers compared two groups of women who were on the same diet plan. The group that also did regular strength-training lost 44 percent more fat than the group that only dieted.

• **Take breaks from your work.** If your work is sedentary (at a desk, for example), get up and move around once an hour or take a short walk in fresh air a couple of times each day. You'll actually save time in the long run because you will work more efficiently.

• **Stretch!** Just a few basic stretches each morning will help to prevent injuries. If you work at a computer, don't forget to stretch your fingers and wrists several times throughout the day, and do shoulder rolls and neck rolls.

4.11 Herbs and Special Supplements

One amazing gift from God is the vast array of medicinal and nutritive plants growing around the world. Throughout the centuries, people have used these to treat an incredible number of injuries, symptoms, and diseases. Chemical analysis has revealed the unique combination of substances in each herb, and scientists are gaining a greater understanding of how these active ingredients affect us.

You'll find many good books on herbal supplements at a bookstore. Since there are an overwhelming number of supplements and herbal preparations, I'm only going to cover what I would consider the most important supplements to keep the immune system healthy, to maintain a healthy cardiovascular system, a healthy musculoskeletal system, and to support body detoxification. Generally, the healthier you are, the fewer supplements you will need. The supplements I am recommending are effective for most individuals to take. Quality is very important when it comes to supplements. Cheaper supplements may lack scientific research and quality controls. Like all things, choose wisely! I have done my homework and the supplements I suggest, and offer, pass rigorous quality standards. This is critical to make sure that products are free of contaminants and to ensure that the dosing meets label claims.

1. A high-quality vitamin supplement. Of course it would be ideal if we could get all of the nutrition we need from the foods we eat daily, but most people have nutritional deficiencies. When we are stressed, eating too fast, or making poor dietary choices, we need to supplement our diet to maintain optimal health. On top of that, many of the foods we eat are depleted of minerals and vitamins because of poor soil conditions and the fact that many fruits are picked prematurely to help extend shelf life. This often contributes to their decreased nutritional value. The better your diet and health is in general the less you will need multivitamins. But regardless, a little additional supplementation can be an important part of prevention.

I am not a fan of taking mega-doses of vitamins and minerals. There are exceptions in certain acute or chronic conditions, but in general I recommend taking conservative amounts. Because I usually have people take less than the label recommends on a multivitamin, most people will not be getting adequate amounts of minerals. Other individuals with sensitive stomachs or absorption issues do better with individual vitamins and minerals. I have also found that most people with candida overgrowth do better (at least during the initial phases of treatment) avoiding B vitamins altogether. Although I have been searching for the ideal multivitamin/mineral/antioxidant that meets everyone's requirements, I have not been successful. My Web site, www.drdyler.com, gives additional guidelines to help you find the ideal regimen for yourself.

2. Extra calcium/magnesium/phosphorous and other bone-building nutrients. Osteopenia and osteoporosis continue to be a problem in the aging population. Adequate calcium starting at childhood, along with weight-bearing exercise, is extremely important for prevention. Supplementing with extra calcium, magnesium, and synergistic bone-building ingredients is especially important for individuals who are not heavy dairy consumers. Of course the amount of supplements needed will depend on dietary consumption, the current state of bone health, how well you digest and absorb nutrients, and the quality of the supplement you are taking. Consult with your health practitioner to determine how much supplementation is right for you and what forms are best for your individual needs. Other nutrients that are critical for building bone include vitamins D, K, C and the minerals phosphorous, boron, and strontium. Most of these can be obtained from a good quality multivitamin, but additional supplementation is often necessary when bone health is already compromised or to avoid overdosing on other nutrients in your multivitamin.

3. A high-quality, stable fish oil product. Research continues to validate the use of fish oils for a host of common health conditions. The fish oil I recommend and use myself is the Eskimo brand. It has been the subject of more than 120 clinical trials and has been proven to reduce cardiovascular disease by reducing cholesterol, increasing the good (HDL) cholesterol, reducing blood pressure, and reducing fibrinogen levels (a protein associated with increased risk of clots). Taking fish oils on a regular basis can reduce symptoms of arthritis and other inflammatory conditions, help delay loss of brain function, increase activity of your body's inherent antioxidant systems, and give your skin a nice healthy glow.

4. Immune support of echinacea. Echinacea has become popular for treating colds, and clinical studies verify that it works. Start taking it at the very first sign of a cold or the flu, or take it every day in small amounts as a lymphatic cleanser. Esberitox®, a popular remedy for the past 70 years in Europe, and more recently in the United States, contains echinacea, baptisia, and thuja and has been proven to shorten the length of the common cold and to boost several different immune parameters. I personally like to take one a day in the winter to help prevent colds. It has been proven safe in children for this purpose as well.

5. Colloidal silver. Although this substance lacks the research of some of the above suggestions, it has been used safely for hundreds of years as a natural anti-microbial substance. I recommend everyone have a bottle in their medicine cabinet to deal with sore throats, coughs, stomach aches, and other symptoms that may be related to minor bacterial infections. Of course this does not replace antibiotics in moderate to severe infections, but when used in conjunction with immune boosters such as echinacea, colloidal silver can often take care of the infection if you catch it early enough. I use colloidal silver concentrated to 30 parts per million which has been shown success in studies (in vitro) to have one of the highest rates of bacterial kill off. One to two tablespoons daily for a week is usually enough to help the body deal with mild to moderate infections.

6. Digestive enzymes. As you get healthier and eat a more balanced diet, your need for digestive enzymes will decrease. Regardless, I would still suggest that enzymes be a part of your regimen because good digestion is the key to health. I currently take enzymes when I eat at restaurants or when I overeat (I try not to but slip occasionally) or when I feel like I'm fighting off a bug. There are enzymes derived from animal sources such as pancreatin, and there are enzymes derived from fungal and plant sources. I tend to use more of the latter enzymes because they operate in a larger pH range and can help digest foods in the stomach all the way down into the large intestine. This can be especially helpful for individuals who are suffering from a large range of food allergies and sensitivities. Some people find pancreatic enzymes more effective for protein digestion, especially when combined with betaine HCl (hydrochloric acid) which can be an added benefit for many individuals. You may want to experiment to see which enzymes best help your particular situation. Enzymes are often prescribed in-between meals as well and act to reduce inflammation within the body. This is useful for athletic injuries and systemic inflammation associated with a variety of health conditions.

7. Body cleansing herbs/detoxification. As you continue to improve your diet and exercise regularly, your need for whole body cleansing will be reduced. However, most adults will benefit from doing a cleanse two to three times a year for a week or two. There are many cleansers available on the market, including colon cleansers with extra fiber and cleansing herbs, liver detoxification products, blood/lymphatic cleansers and candida and parasite cleansers. (See my website for more details.) A health care practitioner, who is knowledgeable in detoxification, can best assist you with your specific detoxification needs. During a cleanse, it is best to follow a somewhat hypoallergenic or simplified diet, which could include rice, steamed vegetables, clear soups, beans, and salads. Dressings should be limited to olive oil, vinegar, and lemon juice, and beverages limited to pure water and herbal teas.

Saunas can be a great way to assist the body in detoxification since the skin is the largest organ of elimination. Many people incorporate clay baths as an additional way of pulling toxins out through the skin. Consult your health care practitioner to see if saunas would be appropriate for you.

Fasting is associated with spiritual matters and should be kept in that light. Even though fasting can have health benefits, I do not recommend it for health reasons as a general rule. It can cause more harm than good, especially in individuals who have a high toxin load. Biblical fasting helps us to draw closer to God and be more tuned in to prayer and God's direction in our lives.

8. Probiotics. Probiotics is a term that refers to the good bacteria, such as lactobacillus and bifido bacteria, often found in yogurt cultures. They are important for your health. These good bacteria form colonies in your intestine and help prevent infection, help produce B vitamins naturally, help further digest food and eliminate waste products, and even have some protective properties against certain types of cancer. Although yogurt contains these active cultures, most of the good bacteria in them will not survive the normal digestive process. Thus, I recommend supplementing with probiotics on a semi-regular basis—definitely after infections or diarrhea, especially if antibiotics were utilized, and also after performing a candida or parasite cleanse. Since these bacteria can and should form colonies of their own in your intestines, it is not necessary to supplement on a daily basis unless there are certain chronic health conditions, such as irritable bowel syndrome, for which that may be appropriate. A product from Japan, Probiotic Pearls, has been shown to be stable through stomach acids and does not require refrigeration.

9. Other considerations. In place of some of those eight glasses of water required each day, incorporate herbal teas into your daily routine.

<u>Therapeutic herbs and foods:</u>

* Green tea is high in flavonoids. Flavonoids have antioxidant properties and, in effect, prevent your "pipes" from "rusting." Green tea contains other active constituents that may be helpful in preventing certain types of cancer as well. A few cups a day can protect your heart and blood vessels. It does contain some caffeine so use in moderation.

* Chamomile soothes upset stomachs. Put two teaspoons of dried chamomile leaves in a cup of boiling water.

* Peppermint tea can be helpful for stimulating digestion after a meal. It has a slight energizing quality without the over-stimulation of caffeine, which makes it a good choice for sensitive individuals.

* Ginger tea benefits digestion and is a natural anti-inflammatory.

For specific health conditions, standardized herbs (herbs that have specific amounts of active ingredients) are the best, because you can be sure that reliable amounts of the active ingredients are in each capsule. Before starting any of these however, make sure that you have incorporated all of the basic fundamentals first including stress reduction, exercise, better diet and the nutritional support listed in numbers 1-8.

* Feverfew can help alleviate migraine headaches. The freeze-dried form is best. The treatment doesn't work right away, but after two months of daily use you should start to feel significantly better. Discontinue use if you don't. Be sure that your doctor has ruled out other possible causes of your headaches first. Butterbur is another herb that has shown beneficial results for reducing migraines.

Dried Berry Extracts:

* Bilberry strengthens tiny capillaries in the eyes, helping to preserve vision.
* Hawthorn berry is excellent for people who are at high risk of developing heart disease, and for people with high blood pressure. Although this is a very safe herb, it shouldn't be taken in combination with heart medications such as digoxin. Take approximately 100 to 200 mg three times a day, in tablet or capsule form. Hawthorn is not a quick fix, but rather something to take every day.
* Elderberry, in liquid extract or tincture form, looks promising for the treatment of flu if you start taking it at the very first sign of symptoms.
* Standardized horse chestnut seed is excellent for uncomfortable varicose veins. It probably works by strengthening the vein walls.

Fresh plants:

* Don't forget garlic! Even though garlic was recently shown

not to improve cholesterol levels, it has shown benefits in reducing atherosclerosis (clotting of arteries) and has natural antibiotic and antifungal properties. Ginger, onions, and turmeric also have many beneficial phytochemicals that can reduce inflammation, support healthy digestion, and add some flavor to your food.

* Aloe plants can be grown at home and used to promote the healing of skin problems. Cut off a leaf, scrape out the gel inside, and apply the gel to eczema, sunburn, minor burns, and acne.

* Four large servings of spinach per week has been useful in the prevention and treatment of macular degeneration, a leading cause of blindness in the central vision.

Other herbs are proving to be very useful, from saw palmetto for prostate, to black cohosh for menopause. Consult with a doctor who is knowledgeable about herbs if you are interested in trying these types of herbal remedies. The *Textbook of Natural Medicine* by Dr. Joseph Pizzorno and Dr. Michael Murray is a great reference book for the researched herbal support protocols for common conditions. You can also visit my Web site at www.drdyler.com for additional information.

Remember, "natural" doesn't always mean healthy or safe. Only use herbs that have been scrutinized for quality control and preferably have positive research associated with them. Don't use them in excessive amounts, and be sure to let your doctor know what you are taking. Some herbs shouldn't be taken in combination with regular medications.

4.12 Common Health Issues

(See my Web site, www.drdyler.com *for a complete list of health conditions)*

1. When Depression Is the Diagnosis

As you begin to understand the Disease Model better, the name given to your illness becomes less and less relevant. Stress, leading to nutritional depletion, or toxicity, leading to a breakdown in your body function—which came first, the chicken or the egg?—all manifest themselves differently, depending on your genetic makeup, or in this case genetic weaknesses. The most important thing is to get the proper diagnosis of what is really going on, *i.e.,* stress, nutritional depletion, toxicity issues, poor dietary or lifestyle choices, and spiritual issues. It is important to have medical and spiritual help, as well as supervision in both diagnosis and treatment of your condition. But neither your doctor nor your pastor or priest is God—the more knowledge you bring to the table, the better off you will be.

Depression is a prime example. Are you depressed because your hormones are out of balance? From lack of sleep? Lack of sunlight? Lack of exercise? A deficiency in protein, which can lead to a decrease in serotonin? Heavy metal toxicity? Is your depression from adrenal or thyroid depletion, or from a lack of community? A lack of purpose? Perhaps you haven't confessed your sins to God and your relationship with Him is suffering. Do you have unresolved anger?

As you can see, the list can go on and on, and that is why it is critical to look at the entire picture. Taking the antidepressants Paxil or Prozac may or may not be appropriate given the actual diagnosis. Certainly taking these drugs without addressing the underlying causes is foolish. If you are already on these drugs, it's not wise to stop them. This must be done slowly under medical supervision if it is the right timing to do so. If you are not on these drugs and are struggling from mild to moderate depression and seeking to understand the cause, there are several natural remedies that may be able to assist you in your overall moods in the interim. Ask your health care practitioner and do some research on your own on the herb St. John's wort, the amino acid tryptophan (which also comes in its active form 5 HTP), or the supplement SAMe. I recommend picking up a copy of the *Textbook of Natural Medicine* by Joseph Pizzorno and Michael Murray. It is an excellent, in-depth reference for individual nutrients and herbs for common conditions.

2. Sleep Disorders

Without a doubt most people in this culture are sleep deprived. Most adults need seven to nine hours of sleep daily. If you can't fit that in during the night, perhaps you can squeeze in a short nap during the day. Even a 30-minute power nap in your car during your lunch hour can do wonders! Unless you get adequate sleep, your body will not be able to efficiently rebuild new tissues, produce adequate hormones or be properly energized.

Occasionally, for whatever reason, everyone is going to toss and turn or be over-stimulated, and sleep poorly. For those nights, a sedative with herbs such as valerian, passion flower, hops and the green tea extract L-theanine can be nice to have on hand. Melatonin, a hormone produced in your brain to begin the sleep cycle, is available over-the-counter as well. Some people do extremely well on low doses of melatonin, whereas others wake up groggy. If you are suffering from mild depression with insomnia, 5-HTP can often improve serotonin levels which in turn can increase melatonin levels naturally.

Serious insomnia will not respond to these gentle treatments. Chronic stress, adrenal fatigue, and an overactive mind can lead to serious sleep disorders that will most likely have to be addressed with stronger medication while the underlying stresses are being resolved. Excessive use of caffeine and stimulants can change the whole adrenal rhythm and make deep sleep unlikely. In women, menopause can contribute to poor sleep and the adrenals (cortisol and DHEA levels) and estrogen/progesterone balance should be assessed. Mental stress and strain and trauma can also induce insomnia and may need temporary treatment with stronger medications along with spiritual and lifestyle counseling. A clear conscience can do wonders for a good night's rest!

3. Weight Loss

Not surprisingly, scientists have discovered a direct link between stress and obesity. Cortisol, a major stress hormone, is a powerful appetite stimulant. The reason for this relates to the fight-or-flight response. The person whose source of stress is an enemy who is chasing him must be able to refuel quickly and frequently to avoid danger or engage in battle. But if this person is stressed out from a hard day at the office, he doesn't need to refuel. He needs to calm down. Unfortunately, his body doesn't realize this. Stress signals the release of cortisol, which keeps the appetite turned to the high position all day long. Stress also causes a surge in insulin, which promotes the storage of fat, particularly in the most dangerous area for heart disease: around the waist. Overweight people, and others who want to be healthy, would be wise to follow all of the recommendations in this book for dealing with stress (see Section 4.14).

I frequently have patients who cannot lose weight because of an underlying metabolic problem. A sluggish liver, thyroid, or adrenal gland can slow progress in this area. Taking your body temperature first thing in the morning before rising is a fairly good assessment of thyroid/adrenal function, in combination with other signs and symptoms. The night before, shake the thermometer down to 93 to 95 degrees Fahrenheit and put it next to your bed. When you wake up, put it under your tongue for five full minutes, moving your body as little as possible during that time. Do this for several mornings in a row. Menstruating women should do this test on the first few days of their menstrual period (to make sure that ovulation temperatures don't interfere with the results). Results averaging less than 97.4 degrees Fahrenheit suggest hypothyroidism, especially if you also have dry skin, sensitivity to cold, fatigue, recurrent infections, and menstrual problems. Try getting an hour of moderately vigorous exercise daily and following the dietary guidelines listed earlier in this section.

You should consult a qualified health practitioner who can help you in these areas. In addition, here are some simple suggestions that many overweight people have found helpful:

1. Be prepared. Recognize that you may encounter many sources of stress throughout the day and that you need to develop a list of strategies that will enable you to respond to the stress with something other than food when your cortisol and insulin levels rise. Literally make a list. For example, if you feel stressed out and have a strong desire to eat something, your list might say: "Pray. Call a friend. Go for a walk. Clean out a closet. Put on a CD and dance." Include whatever is easy, convenient, involving, constructive, and enjoyable for you.

2. Make a plan. You may need to acknowledge that your experience has been that you can't afford to be spontaneous; your split-second food decisions are all too often unhealthy ones. Be sure to plan all of your meals at least 24 hours in advance and don't deviate from the plan. Don't go grocery shopping when you are hungry and always bring a list of the foods that you should buy.

3. Keep it simple. Complicated plans that call for making too many changes in your life usually don't work. At least in the beginning, keep your focus on these five things: exercise, especially walking; increased vegetable consumption; eight cups of water or herbal tea a day; little or no animal fats; and reduction of stress by living and thinking God's way.

4. Discover your triggers. There may be other chemically-induced cravings that science hasn't discovered yet. While the current focus in the media is on carbohydrate cravings, many overweight people have strong cravings triggered by eating saturated fat, or perhaps any kind of fat, especially in combination with simple carbohydrates. In other words, if they were to eat a breakfast of oatmeal, skim milk, and fruit, they may be satisfied until lunchtime. But, if they eat a breakfast of toast with butter and jam, they may have strong cravings for more of these foods that must be satisfied before lunch. Maybe a tuna sandwich with lots of mayonnaise sends you looking for dessert, whereas a salad with low-fat dressing and a plain whole-wheat roll would leave you satisfied. Think carefully about what food triggers, if any, stimulate a powerful desire to eat more. This information will help you plan meals that keep these desires in check.

Another clue to discovering trigger foods is to consider this question: Can you eat only one serving of the food (as defined on the package), or are you virtually incapable of eating only one serving? If you manage to eat only one serving, does it send you off looking for more food immediately or within the hour? These may be signs that you need to eliminate this food completely. Common culprits include white flour, sugar, and foods high in animal fats such as butter, certain cheeses, and mayonnaise.

5. Do something different. Realize that you may need a different plan than you've ever had before. You have probably heard the definition of insanity as doing the same thing over and over, yet expecting a different outcome. How true this is for attempts at weight loss! If using sheer willpower to follow temporary dietary changes hasn't worked for us in the past, only a form of insanity would allow us to think that the same measures will work this time. For example, God's Word doesn't say, "Surround yourself with the things that tempt you, but try really hard not to give in." On the contrary, God usually tells us to flee from temptation, not to go anywhere near it, because He knows how weak we can be. You may need to find ways to avoid contact with the particular foods that trigger cravings for you. That may require: having someone else do the grocery shopping; not watching television anymore to avoid those burger commercials; no longer eating in the cafeteria but instead sitting on a bench outside to eat a meal you've packed; getting rid of cookbooks; clearing out your food cabinets; having someone else in the family put away leftovers; planning meals so that there aren't any leftovers; or having a rule that you'll never eat alone. Find all of the potential food-related pitfalls in your day and make radical changes if you truly want different results this time.

6. Be easy on yourself. If you slip up on your healthy eating routine and devour a whole package of Twinkies, it's okay. Get back on track with your next meal. Don't let the ups and downs of emotions dictate your life and eating habits.

7. Burn off stress. One healthy way to respond to stress is to take a walk. Why? It can trigger the release of feel-good endorphins and burn off the excess cortisol you generated from stress. Both of these factors will counter the effects of cortisol on appetite and fat storage.

8. Get tested for food allergies. Food allergies contribute to sluggish metabolism, elevated stress hormones, and water retention contributing significantly to weight gain. They also contribute significantly to a variety of health issues as described throughout this chapter.

4.13 Anti-aging Programs

As the baby-boomer generation grows older, there is an increasing interest in anti-aging programs. Potent drugs and supplements will be discovered each year in this quest for extending youthfulness. Anti-aging hormone therapies, in particular, have become big business. These are extremely powerful substances, which may be responsible for serious side effects, including emotional imbalance, insomnia, and increased risk of cancer. Before starting any hormones, including estrogen and progesterone, make sure that adequate testing has been done to validate replacement therapy.

Rather than turning to anti-aging hormones and drugs, along with their potential side effects, start with the basic health strategies covered in this chapter. The human body replaces about 300 billion cells per day. If these cells receive adequate nutrition and are not subjected to the damaging effects of stress hormones and toxins, they can be healthier than the ones they replace. Your body contains the most comprehensive pharmacy known to man and just needs the foundational blocks of health to be in place so that it can operate effectively. Following the simple guidelines in this book will reduce stress hormones and support rebuilding and repair mechanisms in the body. Identify and eliminate, if you can, the sources of unnecessary stress in your life. Reorganize your thinking, as described in Chapter 3. Support your body with good nutrition, exercise, and adequate rest. Have interests and help other people. Love others deeply, live in peace whenever possible, laugh freely, and enjoy the good things that God brings your way.

4.14 Stress Reduction Techniques

Check the shelves of your local library or bookstore and you'll discover rows of books on stress reduction, filled with all sorts of tips. If stress was simply a matter of bad habits in our thinking, we'd just pick a few of these tips and live a worry-free life, wouldn't we? In contrast to that, the type of stress reduction that I'm recommending is based on the spiritual awakening described in Chapter 2 and the revolutionary shift in consciousness detailed in Chapter 3. While small stop-worrying tips may still be helpful, the most effective, long-lasting methods will always involve mentally (and sometimes physically) stepping outside of the whirlwind of events and tuning in to God. The foremost way to do this is by reading God's Word. Here are a few more suggestions:

• **Change your first response.** When something happens that upsets you, instead of reacting emotionally, say to yourself, "Stop! How does God see this?" Wait until you have God's wisdom on the situation before speaking or acting. Usually, the world is not waiting on the edge of its seat for our words of wisdom. A hasty response usually isn't necessary. Fretting, being angry, and venting are reactions that, while normal, don't help us reach the solution to our situation. God has the solution! Sometimes He wants us to speak and act; often, He doesn't. Remember that the question isn't just "Is there something here that I can change?" That question must always be accompanied by "Does God want me to change it?" Remember the Serenity Prayer: "God, grant me the serenity to accept the things I cannot change, courage to change the things I can, and the wisdom to know the difference."

• **Pray continually.** Prayer can be a way of being rather than an activity done once or twice a day. Before phoning someone, making a purchase, planning a trip, eating a meal, speaking to your spouse, or disciplining your child, say a prayer. Prayers don't need to be long. For example, as you are about to enter a business meeting or a social gathering, you might stop and ask God's help: "Heavenly Father, please help me to see these people through Your eyes, to act as You would have me act, to care about the people here as You would, and to think before I speak, speaking only the words You would have me say." We have the potential, with God, to eliminate anxiety or feelings of stress, and fearlessly (but meekly) walk into every situation, confident in God's ability to work out absolutely everything for the good. If you want this to be the rule rather than the exception in your life, walk closely with Him, be dependent on Him, listen to Him, and do things His way. If, despite your prayers, you find yourself blurting out statements that you later regret, keep praying. You are a work-in-progress. Our gracious God will forgive you and continue to spend your lifetime helping you to grow spiritually. No time to pray? Rethink this! The more you have to do today, the more you'll need prayer to help you do it the right way.

• **Deep breathing.** When something stressful happens, stop and take a few deep breaths. This will calm your nervous system and give you a chance to reflect instead of reacting emotionally to the situation. Use deep breathing before you pray to pull your mind out of the whirlwind of daily events. Make it a habit to observe your breathing every couple of hours throughout the day in the beginning to monitor how you are doing. Oftentimes a short break, a walk, or a prayer can help to put everything in perspective again.

• **Journaling.** If you enjoy writing or find that it is an effective way for you to sort through feelings, vent, or communicate, journaling is a health-enhancing, stress-reducing tool.

Joshua Smyth of the State University of New York reviewed studies involving more than 800 people. Generally, participants in the studies would write about traumatic events for 20 minutes or so for three days. Immune system function showed improvement, and illness, as reported by the participants, decreased. Smyth conducted a controlled study, reported in the *Journal of the American Medical Association,* which found that patients with mild to moderate asthma and rheumatoid arthritis who wrote for 20 minutes a day for three consecutive days about the most stressful event they had ever experienced had greater reduction in their symptoms four months later compared to those who just wrote about daily plans for 20 minutes each day. Patients in the study didn't particularly enjoy this process; in fact, many of them found it upsetting to write about the assigned topic. James W. Pennebaker of the University of Texas has found that people who wrote about stressful events for 20 minutes a day three to five times a week made half as many visits to the doctor as those who didn't write. It may be that writing affects cortisol production, which, in turn, affects health. Why don't we hear more about these discoveries in the news instead of the latest drug to cure all our ailments?

If you have a relationship with the living God, journaling can become a transformative process, when you incorporate prayer and God's perspective. When you are done writing, examine what you have written in the light of what you know is true from God's Word. For example, you may detect resentment, meanness, criticalness, sarcasm, and other character traits in what you've written, and see a need to take these before God for forgiveness and help in changing. You may realize that a particular problem would not have arisen if you hadn't listened to (or repeated) gossip in the first place, or hadn't been lazy or sought the approval of people rather than God. Start a gratitude journal to help you remember all of the blessings you do have in your life. You will probably be surprised at how many blessings you already have around you and either took for granted or simply overlooked.

• **Weed out stressful activities and clean house!** We can't (and shouldn't) avoid every source of stress; everyday life brings stress of all kinds. But some sources of stress are unnecessary and add nothing to our lives. Look for these and eliminate them if they aren't God-honoring or don't leave you with a feeling of peace. Examples include: competitive games (either as participant or observer); watching the news or reading the newspaper; watching movies and television shows that focus on violence, immorality, or don't match your values or honor God; listening to argumentative radio talk shows; checking your e-mail compulsively throughout the day; and talking on the phone about other people. Examine activities that you feel pressured to do so that others will think well of you.

De-clutter your life! Get organized. Your environment is going to affect your mental well being and your ability or inability to focus on the things that really matter. Clean your closets, filing cabinet, garage, and other junk accumulating areas regularly. Give away your extra clothes, old furniture, and dusty exercise equipment to Goodwill or some other charity organization. You will feel good and someone else will enjoy and utilize them.

• **Relax.** Sometimes, rather than addressing conflicts and problems head-on, it's preferable to take a walk or a long bath so you have a chance to calm down, collect your thoughts, and ask God what to do. It's in vogue now to call virtually everything "spiritual," but a long bath in candlelight is not a spiritual practice; it's a mood enhancer or relaxation technique. Real spirituality involves trusting and obeying God, and drawing close to Him. Just the same, relaxation techniques can play an important role in helping us to slow down and listen to God. Get into the practice of listening to music that praises God. Perhaps you might consider getting a massage or a facial. A walk on the beach can also do wonders. Spiritual retreats are often necessary if you have lost track of the plans and hopes that the Lord has given you. Get into gardening. Learn to play an instrument. Knitting is a great way to relax, develop friendships, and have Bible studies. Sports are beneficial for both men and women to interact, exercise, and have fun. On a nice day, lay in the sun for half an hour while doing some journaling.

• **Consider your conversations.** How much of your time do you spend venting, complaining, arguing, or gossiping? What steps can you take to break these habits? How about fostering healthy relationships instead, encouraging and elevating one another to make good, healthy choices in life? How about mentoring a young person and imparting some of the wisdom you have learned in life?

• **Plan your day with God, and be prepared to throw away your plan.** Is your list of things to do based on what seems urgent, or is it based on God's priorities for your life? Considering Him first will help everything else to fall into place. He has given you enough time to accomplish His will for you today. Put everything before Him without making assumptions. For example, His Word says to attend church, so that is non-negotiable. But being busy with church activities may not be on His agenda for you. Even after you've prayed and believe you know what the Lord wants you to do for the day, look for opportunities to serve Him in the "interruptions." For example, you may need to put aside your plan for the day because someone you know needs help. Or maybe God allows your plans to fall apart because He wants you to turn to

Him for help. Trust God, follow His Word, and remain humble.

A final word of caution: **It is important not to judge others based on their physical health!** Knowing God can make you healthier than you would have been living life your own way, but better health and self-discipline doesn't make you spiritually superior to others. This is completely erroneous thinking. You may be keenly aware of the ways in which you fail to take good care of your body, but you don't know what challenges another person faces, or the path God has laid out for him or her. Please remember, too, that if you have accepted Jesus Christ, God accepts you and loves you completely in your current state of being, whether you munch on chips all day, lounge around watching soap operas, or forget to floss! As you gain knowledge, understanding, wisdom, and strength, undoubtedly you'll make better decisions affecting your health and seek the best for your life, but you'll still make mistakes and have your moments in the valley.

Do not get complacent in your walk with God either. Examine yourself often to see if you have the fruits of the Spirit in your life (see Galatians 5:22-23) or if you are harboring sin. In the context of taking communion, the Bible says, *"So if anyone eats this bread or drinks this cup of the Lord unworthily, that person is guilty of sinning against the body and the blood of the Lord. That is why you should examine yourself before eating the bread and drinking from the cup. For if you eat of the bread or drink the cup unworthily, not honoring the body of Christ, you are eating and drinking God's judgment upon yourself. That is why many of you are weak and sick and some have even died."*[149]

Wow! God takes this sin stuff seriously, doesn't He? He may not care about us eating junk food, but He does care about the state of our heart. As long as we realize that none of us are worthy to drink of the cup and to take the bread and are faithful to confess our sins and turn from them, we will have the right heart attitude before God.

If you are sick and not getting better, you should also seriously consider what is written in the book of James: *"Are any among*

---

[149] 1 Corinthians 11:27-30 New Living Translation

you suffering? They should keep on praying about it. And those who have reason to be thankful should continually sing praises to the Lord. Are any among you sick? They should call for the elders of the church and have them pray over them, anointing them with oil in the name of the Lord. And their prayer offered in faith will heal the sick, and the Lord will make them well. And anyone who has committed sins will be forgiven. Confess your sins to each other and pray for each other so that you may be healed. The earnest prayer of a righteous person has great power and wonderful results."[150]

Good health is a wonderful thing. If you don't have it, however, be patient and continue to seek for answers and for healing. Remember, from God's eternal perspective, we spend a very short time in our bodies, and physical health is a temporary concern. Someday, if you have a relationship with the living God, you will have a spiritual body and live in God's presence. If you look back on your life here on earth, you wouldn't be concerned about youthfulness, saturated fat, sexuality, or physical fitness. You'd be more likely to consider: "Did the people around me know how much I loved them? Did I let them know how much God loves them? Did I give my all to serving God, to glorifying Him and praising Him by how I lived my life?"

---

[150] James 5:13-16

CHAPTER 5

One Day at a Time

I t is my prayer for you and for myself that we not miss out on any good and perfect gift that comes down from our Father in heaven (see James 1:17).

Happy is the person who finds wisdom and gains understanding. For the profit of wisdom is better than silver, and her wages are better than gold. Wisdom is more precious than rubies; nothing you desire can compare with her. She offers you life in her right hand, and riches and honor in her left. She will guide you down delightful paths; all her ways are satisfying. Wisdom is a tree of life to those who embrace her; happy are those who hold her tightly.[151]

Wouldn't it be a shame if we were distracted by things, even good things that have little or no eternal value, that rob us of time and energy at the expense of what could have been? Lord, may it not be so!

If you are overwhelmed by the number of changes you want to make in your life or you are feeling like it is too late for you to fix

---

[151] Proverbs 3:13-18 New Living Translation

up your life, slow down! Remember, God's timing is perfect for all things and He doesn't ask you to do more than you can handle in His strength, one day at a time. Healing is a journey and it takes time.

The key is to stay tuned in to God. As I have said throughout these chapters, God's ways for us are simple—if we diligently seek Him and His will for our lives. No complicated formulas to master, diets to follow, or exercises to do. God is the author and finisher of our faith, and it is by His Spirit that we can live out the impossible life He is calling us to. Over time, He will mold and shape us so that when He uses us as His instruments we will make a beautiful sound.

So if you mess up, get up, confess your sins, and begin a new day in the refreshment of His love, grace, and mercy. *"The unfailing love of the LORD never ends! By his mercies we have been kept from complete destruction. Great is his faithfulness; his mercies begin afresh each day. I say to myself, 'The LORD is my inheritance; therefore I will hope in him.' "*[152]

Above all, make your life worth living by seeking the happiness that comes with knowing God personally. Living God's way in relationship with Him can greatly reduce your stress levels. After all, you were created to love and enjoy God and live completely dependent on Him. Your mind, body, and spirit were specifically designed to fulfill that purpose. That is the fundamental truth against which the ego so furiously rebels. When we are yoked to God, walking in step with Him, we will have peace. When we don't, we won't. The natural result of walking without Him or out of step with Him is to experience fear, anxiety, restlessness, unease, depression, dissatisfaction, confusion, anger, or irritability—in a word, stress.

Once again, stress is also reduced when we change how we perceive sources of stress and how we react to them. We do have a choice, and, if we have a relationship with God, we have help. Certainly, the death of a spouse/loved one or a severe illness will be stressful to virtually everyone and out of our control. These

---

[152] Lamentations 3:22-24 New Living Translation

types of pains may never be fully healed on this side of heaven and need to be sacrificially given to the Creator when the pains flare up. But most stressful experiences are not as intense. They are your everyday, run-of-the-mill stresses, which cumulatively take their toll on our health and sense of well-being. These experiences, however, are not necessarily stressful in and of themselves. It is our perception of the experience that determines whether or not it is stressful. For example:

- Two people are suffering from chronic health issues; one searches for answers and sees a health professional to confront the problem, the other is worried he has something serious and avoids going to get help at all.
- Two people are hired to run intense sales departments; one is energized and excited, the other is overwhelmed.
- Two people find that a strange insect has invaded their gardens; one is curious and begins research to solve the problem, the other frets over her tomatoes and her day is ruined.
- Two people meet a woman who is competitive and condescending; one goes home to pray for her, the other spends hours in imaginary arguments with this irritating person.

Knowing God can bring peace in even these everyday occurrences, from the traffic jam to the snide neighbor. Not because we complacently say, "Oh, whatever," when anything happens, but because we learn more and more to look at each experience as an opportunity to be faithful to God, and as a chance to see the amazing things that He does.

As long as we are alive on this earth the lessons of life will continue and we will have the opportunity to choose how to respond. The happiest people will generally be the ones who, more often than not, stop to pray or to consider things from God's perspective. They view this as God's universe, not their own. They view life as part of God's plan, rather than measuring every person or event against their own grand plan. They ask God, "How can I be faithful to You in this small (or large) situation? How can I serve You? How can I glorify You? How can I obey You? How do You see this person, Lord, and how do You want me to see him? What are You teaching me in this trial, or through this person?"

The answer will not always be immediately apparent. Perhaps we are being asked to trust God and wait patiently. Rather than irritation, He may desire cheerfulness, helpfulness, quietness, or an action that changes a situation. Sometimes we are being taught a lesson we might not be eager to learn: loss of pride, deepened humility, less reliance on money for our security, to remain silent rather than advising or arguing. The lesson may simply be that God knows what is best for us, even if all we feel at the moment is pain, rejection, or loneliness.

Making God's Word part of our very being will equip us in all of our experiences to see things His way. God's Word becomes part of us through daily reading, meditating on His Word, praying over His Word, being taught by other believers, and Scripture memorization. When we have the sense of peace that comes only from knowing the living God, we do not experience life in the same way. Seeing life through God's eyes revolutionizes our perspective, our relationships, and our reactions, leading to ease, rather than dis-ease, in mind, body, and spirit.

Growing in Knowledge of God

As we know Jesus better, his divine power gives us everything we need for living a godly life. He has called us to receive his own glory and goodness! And by that same power, he has given us all of his rich and wonderful promises. He has promised that you will escape the decadence all around you caused by evil desires and that you will share in his divine nature.

So make every effort to apply the benefits of these promises to your life. Then your faith will produce a life of moral excellence. A life of moral excellence leads to knowing God better. Knowing

God leads to self-control. Self-control leads to patient endurance, and patient endurance leads to godliness. Godliness leads to love for other Christians, and finally you will grow to have genuine love for everyone. The more you grow like this, the more you will become productive and useful in your knowledge of our Lord Jesus Christ.[153]

The celestial sky symbolizes (inadequately, of course) the reality of the glory of God. Without the sun (Jesus) there is no life. The moon (mother, Mary) reflects brilliantly the glory and power of the sun. The stars (you and I) make up the vastness of the sky, and when combined tell an even bigger story of the magnificent Artist Creator's love for humanity.

"Let your light so shine before men, that they may see your good works, and glorify your Father which is in heaven."[154]

For more information and further support on your journey towards optimal health go to www.drdyler.com.

---

[153] 2 Peter 1:3-8 New Living Translation
[154] Matthew 5:16 King James Version

Printed in the United States
200104BV00005B/130-171/A